Dear Laura,

Happy Read...

Love, Brooke

Not Another Diet Book

"As our new age moves forward, more and more people are making sophisticated choices about their health care, with their doctors as *guides*, not gods. It is in keeping with this new principle of self-responsibility that greater numbers of people are looking beyond the immediate goal of *obtaining* their desired weight, to lifestyle changes that will allow them to maintain and sustain that weight. Through Reflective Relearning (a process of contacting the subconscious mind) you can learn to obtain, maintain, and sustain your desired weight for life — with *you* at the helm, directing the process and getting what you want . . ."

— *From the book* —

I tried every diet that I could find — without success. For 37 years, I went through the same cycle of depriving myself, only to gain *more* weight after each attempt. When I heard Dr. Sommer on T.V., I was desperate enough to push aside my doubts. I thought, *this makes sense: I don't need to diet —I need to change my life style!* I put Dr. Sommer's six-week program into practice. Now, 14 months and 48 pounds later, I *know* that I will never be fat again. But even more exciting is the assurance that I have the power to make things happen in my own life.

— *D.O., Colton, CA* —

About The Author

Bobbe L. Sommer, Ph.D., was born and raised in Kansas City. She attended the University of Colorado at Boulder, becoming first an elementary school teacher and later a school psychologist. After receiving a Master's degree from California State University at Los Angeles, she became a psychology instructor at several Southern California community colleges. She received her doctorate in psychology in 1980 and branched out from education to develop a career as a psychological consultant and motivational speaker.

Through her research and private practice, Dr. Sommer has gained an understanding of the factors that keep people from obtaining and maintaining their desired weight. She shares these insights in her workshops, lectures, and books, and is a popular radio and television personality, regularly giving lecture tours all across the country. Her lecture topics include family and daily living, teacher education, weight management, positive lifestyles and self-improvement. She has led seminars for a wide range of organizations, including the California State Universities, numerous corporations, business and professional associations, and women's groups.

Dr. Sommer is a licensed Marriage, Family and Child Counselor. She has also served as a staff and consulting psychologist for various weight clinics. She is a member of, among others, the American Association of Marriage, Family and Child Counselors, the American Association of Sex Educators, Counselors and Therapists, the Foothill Association of School Psychologists, the Harbor Clinical Hypnotherapy Association, and the National Speakers' Association.

She lives with her husband, Charles, and their three sons in San Clemente, California, in a hillside home overlooking the ocean. In addition to this book, she has published two motivational programs on audio cassettes, and is the author of *Never Ask a Cactus For a Helping Hand,* and *The Facts Behind Your Figure.*

Not Another Diet Book

A RIGHT-BRAIN PROGRAM FOR SUCCESSFUL WEIGHT MANAGEMENT

Bobbe Sommer, Ph.D.

Hunter House

Grateful acknowledgement is given for permission to reprint copyrighted tables in Appendix I from *Left Brain, Right Brain* by Sally P. Springer and Georg Deutsch, published by W. H. Freeman and Company, ©1981.

Library of Congress Cataloging-in-Publication Data:

Sommer, Bobbe L.
    Not Another Diet Book.

    1. Reducing — Psychological aspects. 2. Self-help
        techniques
1. Title.
RM222.2.S656   1987   613.2'5   86-7274
ISBN 0-89793-046-0
ISBN 0-89793-037-1 (paperback)

Manufactured in the United States of America

9 8 7 6 5 4 3 2   First edition

Published in 1987 by
   House Inc., Publishers
   P.O. Box 1302,
   Claremont, CA 91711
   U.S.A.

Distributed in Canada by
   N.C. Press
   P.O. Box 4010, Station A
   Toronto, M5W 1H8
   CANADA

Distributed in U.K. by
   Momenta Publishing Ltd.
   Broadway House, The Broadway,
   Wimbledon, London SW 19
   ENGLAND

Book and cover design by Qalagraphia
Editing by Chris Moose
Cover and interior illustrations by Gary Oliver
Incidental line art by Paul Frindt
Color separations by American Lithographic Impression
Set in 11 on 12 point Goudy Olde Style by Richmond House

Contents

Preface

To The Reader

This is definitely NOT another DIET book. As a matter of fact, this is probably an "anti-diet" book. This book presents, first of all, a philosophy, and, second, a practical formula to follow.

The philosophy is a simple one: *Weight is in consciousness.* That is, our bodies reflect what we hold in our thoughts and in our minds. It follows, therefore, that weight management begins with how we think.

The practical formula is a step-by-step, day-by-day procedure to follow for six weeks. I call it Reflective Relearning. If you follow this program, I promise that you will see significant, positive results in your weight.

Recently, a television interviewer asked me if Reflective Relearning *really* works. I told him that it does, indeed, work, as a matter of fact, I would guarantee that it works — unfortunately, I cannot guarantee that the *person* will work.

This book is for all of you who are, as the cover suggests, overwhelmed by the latest fad diets. There are hundreds of these diets which suggest that we can shed unwanted weight virtually within minutes: "The Bees' Knees and Poached Gnats Eggs Diet," "How I Lost 17 Pounds in 2 Hours," and "How I Lived on Brussels Sprouts for 15 Years."

While the diets you have tried may not have names or promise results that are *quite* as farfetched as these, most fad diets are equally ridiculous, ineffective, and sometimes downright dangerous to your health.

They don't work because the old pressures and patterns of thoughts and feelings that are behind weight problems still remain. As soon as the diet is over, these old patterns rise up again and the weight comes back.

This is the book you have been waiting for, and it is NOT ANOTHER DIET BOOK!

Bobbe Sommer
San Clemente, 1986

Acknowledgments

A book like this is never the work of a single person. I owe thanks to many, many people with whom I have come into contact in my private practice, workshops and lectures. They have all contributed to my understanding of the issues involved in weight management, and with their help I have developed the techniques of Reflective Relearning that are the heart of this book.

I want to express my particular appreciation to the following:
— To Barbara Ardinger, Ph.D., my thanks for the rewrites and research that you did so well.
— To Kiran Rana, my publisher, thank you for having faith in my work and for your valuable editorial insights.
— To Chris Moose, my editor, for your ability to re-express what I wanted to say — thanks!

IMPORTANT NOTICE

The material in this book is primarily for educational purposes. The author neither diagnoses problems nor prescribes specific remedies. Any program of diet and exercise should be undertaken after consulting your doctor. Those who embark on such a program on their own, which is their right, must take full responsibility.

This book is dedicated to my family:

Chuck, Rob, Charles, Chris & "Smokie"
— thanks for being uniquely you!

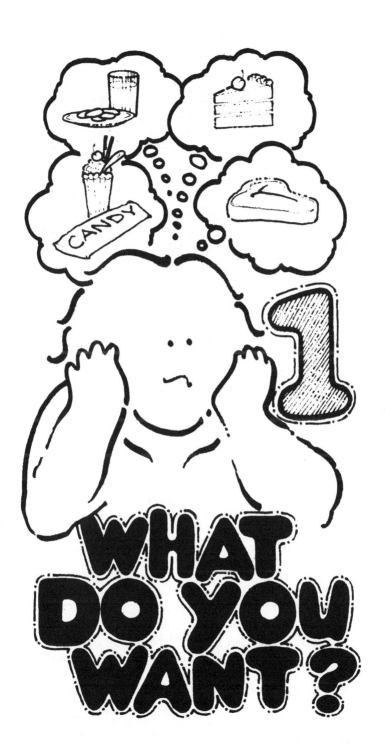

FOR MORE THAN A DECADE, I have worked in a wide variety of weight clinics and have participated in many different types of weight programs — as a clinic director, as a counselor, and as a consulting psychotherapist. The people with whom I have worked include men and women, homemakers and business exectives, teachers and lawyers, assembly line workers and civil servants. They have ranged in age from eight to eighty. Yet they have all had one thing in common: They were among the seventy million people in the United States who were clinically obese. In plain old everyday terms, they were fat. And they were suffering from all the emotional and physical anguish that term implies. This book is dedicated to them and to everyone who is experiencing the pain of being overweight.

I didn't start out as a weight "expert." (Who *starts* as an expert in anything?) Rather, my work with overweight people began serendipitously. I was teaching courses in self-hypnosis for pain control at a university in Los Angeles when a couple of physicians heard me speak. They were involved in a weight clinic and asked me whether the principles I was teaching would apply to weight control. I responded that they would, and the physicians then asked whether I would be interested in participating in a weight loss clinic that they wanted to establish.

I confided that I was definitely not interested in aversion therapy — where people are electrically shocked or otherwise harassed in an attempt to change their behavior. I also stated that I was not interested in the pills and shots sometimes used to assist people who were obese. The doctors assured me that they were starting a modified fasting program — in which people would be restricted to a very few calories daily, and would be supervised by physicians to make it as safe as possible. The doctors were interested in my becoming the psychological director of the weight loss clinic.

I still felt some "gut level" hesitation to become involved in a weight *loss* program — an intuitive hanging back. For some time, I had been interested in the research of Dr. Roger Sperry and his colleagues on the functions of the right and left hemispheres of the brain. The research had made me aware of the importance of the right brain as the intuitive, holistic, visionary partner to the intellectual, analytical, left brain. As a result, I had learned to listen to the valuable "right-brain" part of me. After our first meeting I told the physicians that I wanted to go home and reflect upon their proposal.

When I got up the next morning, I went into my walk-in closet (the only quiet spot in my home of three active teenage boys) and began to do my "Reflective Relearning" exercises — a meditative program which I use daily to "tune in" to my right-brain intuitions. Sitting in that walk-in closet was my way of getting in touch with my silent partner, my right brain. By repeating "OM, OM, OM," to myself, over and over, I was able to allow my analytical, logical, left-brain thoughts to subside while I called up my intuitive, emotional, right-brain response to the situation confronting me. *I was putting my conscious awareness (my left brain) in touch with what my subconscious, "hidden" thoughts and images (my right brain) had to say.*

As I was "oming" away, I began to reflect upon the doctors' proposal. Why was I feeling resistance toward it? What part of their presentation didn't sit well with me? Suddenly, a gigantic red "O" appeared in my mind's eye. It gradually elongated to spell out OBTAIN. Now, although this image meant nothing to my logical mind, I persevered. Those of us who practice this form of meditative "thinking" have learned to take what we get!

I continued repeating "OM, OM, OM," and soon a large red "M" appeared and elongated to spell out MAINTAIN. Then, spontaneously, my eyes flew open and I "got" the message. My left brain grasped what my right brain and subconcious mind were communicating to me. I knew then that I didn't want to participate in a weight *loss* program. I didn't (and don't) believe that people are "losers." Instead, I wanted to teach people how to *obtain* and *maintain* their desired weight.

When I gained this insight into why I felt resistance at the words "weight loss," I shared my new awareness with the physicians. They agreed that we would emphasize obtaining and maintaining desired weight and focus upon a more positive avenue to weight control. Later, as I worked with groups of overweight people, we added the term *sustain* to this formula to underscore the notion of an ongoing, lifetime program. Thus was born the OMS method: Obtain, Maintain, and Sustain your desired weight — for life.

NO BLAMING OR SHAMING

When I began to work as a weight counselor, I had to explore my own prejudices concerning "fat people." Did I harbor feelings of disgust toward them? Did I have any hidden belief that they were fat because they were just too lazy to control their weight? Did the fact that I had never been more than ten pounds over my desired weight make it impossible for me to understand the pain they were experiencing? I knew I had to face the issue of whether I *blamed* these people for being overweight.

In asking myself these questions and in conducting group sessions with more and more overweight people, I began to discern some interesting, nearly universal patterns. Countless men and women were saying the same thing about their weight. I learned from hundreds of people that they became fatter after each unsuccessful diet. I learned that being fat means having to be "jolly" and a "good guy" to compensate for the fear of being rejected by others. Most of all, I learned that being fat is feeling out of control — perhaps the most threatening feeling a human being can experience. These people were revealing horror stories of eating and crying simultaneously. They told of consuming huge amounts of food in the closet and hiding ice cream cartons at the bottom of the garbage can. *I learned that fat is not the issue. The issue is feelings — the terrible pain that overweight people deal with daily in their battle of the bulge.*

I knew then that what I felt for these people was compassion and empathy. I also knew that I wanted to dedicate much of my time to learning about eating behavior and teaching others to gain control over food. And I was convinced, more than ever, that diets and pills and the "just push yourself away from the table" approach would never work. From hundreds of hours of running weight therapy groups, I discovered that those of us who are overweight must take control of our LIVES if we are to take control of our eating habits.

Where and how to start seemed an insurmountable task at first, but the groups taught me well. They taught me that dealing with fat merely at the intellectual level cannot work. It is like trying to put out a raging fire with a small bucket of water —

sometimes the hand that isn't throwing the water on the fire is fanning the flames! That is exactly what happens when we concentrate on what only half of our brain — the intellectual, reasonable, left half — tells us, and ignore what the emotional, intuitive, right half has to say. Our society tends to put down what cannot be explained logically. We have learned to ignore half of our thinking, so it's no wonder that this half-brained approach often ends up in ineffective, self-destructive results. Where weight is concerned, this tendency translates into "Just reduce your caloric intake, and you'll lose weight." True enough — but *not* enough. In order to change our lives, we must change our thoughts, and only when we learn to use all of our brain, not just half of it, can we do that.

TWO BRAINS ARE BETTER THAN ONE

The notion of getting in touch with our right brain may seem like hocus-pocus to some, but to me it is very important. Granted, the process may be hard to understand — logically, with the left brain. "And what in the world," you may well ask, "does all this right-brain stuff have to do with me grabbing a candy bar whenever I'm upset?" Good question — and one we need to address here and now. I'm going to start by talking to your left brain — your logical, analytical, rational side, the side all of us have learned to trust. There is reliable, empirical evidence substantiating the "illogical" yet essential functioning of the right brain and the profound influence it has on our behavior. So let's take a quick "minicourse" in brain and mind, or "what you've been dying to know about your right brain, but your left brain was too afraid to ask."

Though the brain in your head is a single mass of tissue, the right and left cerebral hemispheres actually make up a double organ, which is joined together by a band of nerve fibers called the *corpus callosum.* (A "map" of the brain is provided in Appendix I.) Although physiologically the two halves of the brain are mirror images of each other, scientific research has shown that in function they differ greatly from each other.

Evidence of this dual functioning has been around for a long time, but the real breakthrough in research came in the 1960s, when Dr. Roger Sperry and his students Michael Gazzaniga and Jerre Levy began their historic split-brain experiments. In these experiments they were able to test the independent thinking abilities of two surgically separated halves of a brain, and they discovered some pretty amazing things. They found that each half of the brain has its own special train of thought and its own memories. Even more important, they found that the two sides of the brain think in fundamentally different ways. While the left brain tends to think in words, the right brain thinks in sensory images. That is, for the vast majority of people, the left brain controls language functions — the production and comprehension of speech — whereas the right brain thinks in pictures, like the ones I saw when I was meditating on my possible involvement with a weight "loss" clinic. Furthermore, the right brain seems to excel in spatial abilities, or the recognition of how things relate three-dimensionally, in space. It is that ability which allows us to put on our clothes, move from room to room and recognize faces — in short, to form, store, and respond to pictorial images that mean something to us.

If you have ever known a person who has suffered a stroke to one side of the brain, you will know what I mean. Left-brain-damaged stroke patients can recognize the faces of friends and relatives, but they often slur their words or have absolutely no ability to understand or produce speech (depending on the extent of the brain damage). Right-brain-damaged patients, on the other hand, are able to understand what is said to them and respond articulately, but when it comes to putting on a bathrobe, getting to the bathroom, or even recognizing their visitors, they are often at a loss.

Perhaps one of the most intriguing differences in right- and left-brain functions has to do with emotions. Stroke patients who have sustained damage to the right cerebral hemisphere are often unable to interpret or respond to the "nonverbal language" of others, as may be expressed in a raised eyebrow, an angry tone of voice, or a shrug of the shoulders. Moreover, these patients seem to have difficulty expressing emotions — they seem to have lost

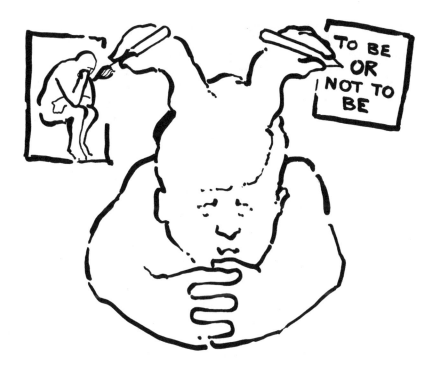

While the left brain tends to think in words, the right brain thinks in sensory images — in pictures.

touch with their feelings.

There are various schools of thought concerning what, exactly, causes these functions of our "two" brains to be different, but most people agree that the abilities of our two cerebral hemispheres are equally essential to a full human existence. Most also agree that the left brain is responsible for the verbal, logical, analytical, intellectual, deductive, abstract aspect of our thinking, while the right brain is the seat of our visuo-spatial, holistic, intuitive, sensuous, imaginative, concrete "thoughts."

I place "thoughts" in quotation marks because most of us would describe thoughts as ideas we express in words in our heads, silently rather than aloud. It is now clear, however, that the right brain also has thoughts; we simply neglect to recognize them as such because they are not expressed in words until they are communicated (via the *corpus callosum*) to the left brain and translated into language. Perhaps it would be wise to recall the old Chinese adage, "A picture is worth a thousand words." The right brain does have thoughts of its own. They are expressed in images and emotions, and they affect our behavior every day of our lives, whether we know it or not.

THE BRAIN-MIND NEXUS

Next, let's take a look at how the conscious and subconscious minds work. The idea of "mind" is just that — an idea, a theory. There is no anatomical part of the body called THE MIND. Rather, it is an abstract concept that is variously identified with personality, memory, "the essence of me," self-identity, even "spirit" or "soul." Many psychologists have defined "mind" as "consciousness," with the unconscious, the subconscious, and the conscious as the three components of that consciousness.

The unconscious mind comprises memory traces so deeply buried that, for all intents and purposes, they no longer exist within us. For that reason, the unconscious does not concern us here. It is the subconscious and the conscious minds that we can work with to modify our thinking and behavior.

The conscious mind is the one with which we are most familiar. It works at the awareness level, setting goals and making decisions. It "speaks" to us, usually in words, telling us not to forget to buy the milk when we go to the store or to be sure to take that red silk dress to the dry cleaner's before next week's party. The conscious mind "knows" what's going on in our normal waking state. It decides it wants or needs something and sets to work to get it. It is critical and evaluative; it may tell you that "that was a dumb thing to say" or that a movie was good because the special effects were sensational.

The subconscious mind, on the other hand, does not work at the awareness level. It doesn't make decisions. Instead, it follows the mandates of the conscious mind, acts upon its demands, and mediates the creative process of bringing about end results. Eventually, many things that were once in your conscious mind are relegated to the subconscious realm, since they have become far too simple for the conscious mind to bother with. Do you remember the first time you drove a car? Did you drive it consciously? You bet you did! You carried on a running conversation with yourself: "Now step on the gas, oops, slow down, touch the brake, turn the wheel, that's too much...". But now, more experienced, you have relegated almost all driving to your "automatic pilot," the subconscious mind. Only under unusual circumstances does the conscious mind take control again, as when a large truck suddenly pulls in front of you. You *consciously* attend to that situation! Of course, your subconscious mind has already slammed your foot on the brake, but your consciousness is very much on that truck and nothing else until the danger has passed.

Let's take another example. Right now, quickly cross your legs. Okay, which leg is on top? You had a choice, you know, but did you consciously think about which leg to cross over? Few of us do. Your subconscious mind heard the command and crossed one leg (probably the right) over the other without "you" having to think about it.

Unlike the conscious mind, the subconscious is completely noncritical and nonjudgmental. It simply attends to the needs of the consciousness with "automatic" responses that have been stored in its databank of problem-solving mechanisms. Although we are rarely "aware" of its presence, it is constantly at work just below the level of consciousness, helping us deal with our daily lives.

Sometimes, if we fail to attend to our subconscious (as when we fail to attend to a problem at work that we know will eventually have to be solved), the subconscious will "scream" its message to us via a dream — often a nightmare. Indeed, dreams, daydreams, and fantasies are among the many naturally occurring *altered states of consciousness* through which our subconscious mind communicates directly with our consciousness. I will have more to say about such altered states later, for they are the avenues whereby we can become aware (conscious) of how our subconscious affects our behavior. By putting ourselves in touch with the workings of the subconscious, we can learn to reprogram our subconscious thoughts in order to redirect our behavior.

If we were to draw a diagram of the right and left hemispheres of the brain and superimpose it on a map of the conscious and subconscious minds, which parts would align themselves? As you probably suspect, the right brain and the subconscious mind tend to work together, while the left brain and the conscious mind tend to correlate. The right brain thinks visually, holistically, synthetically, nonevaluatively — characteristics it shares with the subconscious mind. The left brain thinks in symbols (words and numbers), step by step (sequentially), analytically, and critically — characteristics also associated with the conscious mind. We literally, then, have *two kinds of thinking in one head!*

"So what does all of this have to do with me and my weight?" you may still be asking. The answer is simple: A deeper understanding of how the right brain and the subconscious mind affect our behavior will open the door for many of us to change that behavior. Only with this understanding can we get to our desired weight and *stay* there. Indeed, such understanding is imperative. The implications of both the subconscious mind and the right brain for the control of eating behavior have been severely neglected.

Many health professionals have taken the stand that all you need to do to "lose" weight is push yourself away from the table and eat less. Their approach usually consists of handing the patient a good diet and telling him to stick to it. Along with it they hand out a few good lines, like: "Fewer calories equals weight reduction." "Eat less, weigh less." "Here, follow this diet and exercise regularly and you'll reach your weight goal in a year."

The left-brain logic of such formulas is impeccable. If only our logical left brain controlled our eating behavior, the approach would work just fine. Unfortunately, as we all know, this approach isn't fine at all: The more we force ourselves to stick to the regimen, the less "fine" we feel. If we slip, we feel silly, out of control, and helpless, because we know that it is only a matter of time before we fall off the wagon altogether and become even worse "failures" than we were before. Even when we do manage to "lose" enough to reach our weight goal, few of us have thought beyond that goal to how we will *maintain* that desired weight. So we return to old habits, overeating to reward ourselves for the deprivation we've suffered. Sound familiar? For most of us, this left-brain-only approach to weight management — whether it takes the form of constant dieting, pill-taking, or even surgery — can never work. All it does is engage us in a continuing up-down battle, a battle with ourselves. It is now time to consider the part of ourselves that we have been fighting: the right brain, the subconscious mind. As you will learn in this book, the right brain's intuitive knowledge is essential in nearly all facets of our lives, and we are long overdue in exploring how to tap its power within us. The OMS method, which is described in this book, utilizes the functions of the right brain and the subconscious mind in a process called Reflective Relearning. Through this process, outlined later in this book, you will learn to use *all* of your brain and *all* of your mind to obtain, maintain, and sustain your desired weight for life.

WEIGHT IS YOUR CHOICE

That is what the OMS method of Reflective Relearning is all about: changing our lives. Its premise is this: *Weight is in consciousness.* By this I mean that weight is a function of thought — or, to be more precise, weight is a function of a behavior that results from a thought. Thought, in turn, is a product of *all* of the brain, the right as well as the left. To speak in terms of the mind, weight is a function of both the subconsciousness and the consciousness.

If there is a "trick" to the OMS method, it is this: *We must bring our subconscious, right-brain thoughts and drives to consciousness, harmonizing them with our left-brain thoughts, in order to bring about behavioral change.* We can change nothing in our lives until we bring our knowledge from the subconscious to the conscious level. How can we break habits of which we are unaware? We have all had the experience of learning from others about a behavior that annoys them. Usually we are *un*-conscious that our behavior is offensive. Once we become conscious that cracking peanuts in bed makes our mate climb the walls, we can make a choice to change the irritating habit — or drive our mate out of the bed.

That's the good news: *Your body weight is your choice.* And there is no bad news! Sure, there are those who say that being overweight is biologically and hereditarily determined. They would argue that you simply inherited a bunch of "fat genes" that are programmed to stay fat forever. There are others who claim that being overweight is an emotional disorder that needs to be treated with psychotherapy. Another school sees intellectual (left-brain) understanding and insight into our behavior as all we need to control our eating.

These theories are certainly valid — as far as they go. For example, there is no doubt that some of us have a genetic predisposition toward becoming obese. Likewise, there are some obese individuals who would benefit from psychotherapy. It is also true that cognitive (left-brain) insight into why overeating makes us gain weight is extremely helpful in changing that behavior. Nevertheless, all of these theories approach weight control only from a logical, left-brain perspective. They disregard the subtle functions of the right brain and the subconscious mind, which must be brought into play if people are to get to their desired weight and, more important, alter their lifestyles in order to *keep* that weight. We must learn how half of our brain — the neglected right half — has come to regard food and eating. Once we have learned that, we can begin to bring our two brains into alignment and learn new ways, or relearn, older, healthier ways of behaving that will enable us to obtain, maintain, and sustain our desired weight for life.

Note: I do not advocate "dieting" in this book, nor do I talk about your "ideal" weight — what is ever "ideal"? The term sounds lovely, but it connotes something entirely unobtainable, rather like Utopia. This book outlines specific, practical ways for you to choose and keep your *desired* weight, the weight at which you feel optimally healthy, both physically *and* emotionally.

First, we will explore some traditional (and, unfortunately, still current) approaches to weight control — diets, pills, and surgery —

to see what they have to offer and where they can go wrong. Next, we will look at ways that brain and mind functions have affected our behavior in the past, so that we can become aware of how we gained unwanted fat in the first place. Finally, you will learn how to use the brain-mind-consciousness connection, step by step, not only to reach your desired weight but also to keep that weight. For those who choose to embark on this Reflective Relearning program, two appendices list sources for further information on brain and mind functions and the basics of good nutrition.

The book will allow you to gain both an intellectual, left-brain understanding of the processes described and attain right-brain insights via the experiential, "how-to" material in Chapters 6, 7 and 8. By means of the Reflective Relearning exercises presented in those chapters, you *can* begin, right now, to move toward your desired weight.

Remember, you can change your mind. Where is it written that you have to be fat forever? The OMS method of Reflective Relearning is no panacea; it is not a definitive answer to all weight challenges. But it has worked for thousands of people who have applied its principles on a daily basis. You may at first wonder how it can work. It is, after all, subtle, simple, experiential, nonintellectual — something the left brain finds difficult to accept because it draws on an aspect of knowingness that we have ignored for years, perhaps for a lifetime. Yet it does work.

It works if you do it. Remember, when you and I are feeling FULFILLED, we tend not to FILL FULL. When we allow ourselves to go after what we want (our desired weight), we begin to commit ourselves to reaching and keeping that goal, which is, after all, just another way of saying that we take responsibility for our actions. We have made a *choice*.

You can allow yourself to replace filling full with fulfillment through the OMS method of Reflective Relearning. You have nothing to lose and everything to gain: the weight you want and the life you want. Think it over. What *do* you want? Make the choice, take the responsibility. Then read on and enjoy the experience.

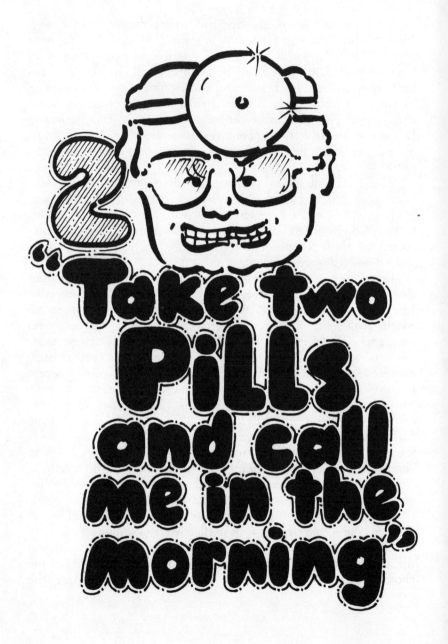

2

"Take two Pills and call me in the morning"

GOING ON A DIET, BY POPULAR DEFINITION, implies that I am going to "starve," or at least deprive myself for a given time, until I reach a desired goal-weight. Thus defined, a diet is also a sure-fire road to failure. Psychologically, whenever we deprive ourselves of something for a given period of time, we soon expect to reward ourselves for a job well done. Remember, for the majority of people, dieting is a much-hated experience, to be endured only temporarily. When the goal is achieved, it's back to old, comfortable habits. And that's the Catch-22 for most of us. We simply do not plan past the end of the diet.

It is important to recognize this fact now, at the beginning of this book, since dieting is fast becoming an American way of life. Everybody talks about his or her diet, usually the latest fad diet. Take away those new, exciting, ever-promising diets, and what's left to talk about at a cocktail party?

Our emphasis in this book, however, is away from the concept of diets. Instead, we will focus on a long-term dedication to changing lifestyle adaptive patterns. What are "lifestyle adaptive patterns"? Quite simply, they are the behaviors we have formed for coping with our day-to-day lives, particularly our emotions. For too many of us this has meant dieting, depriving, and rewarding, which leads to an emotional merry-go-round of lost and regained pounds.

In order to change these lifestyle adaptive patterns, we must learn to incorporate different *thinking* patterns into our daily behavior. We must learn to think of going for a walk or taking a warm shower instead of eating when we are frustrated, angry, bored, excited, or whatever. When we do not think of how to handle these emotions, we go back to our old, habitual adaptive patterns. Through past conditioning, many of us have learned to "adapt to," or handle, unpleasant situations through the use of food. As you will see when you read Chapters 3 and 4, many of us have subconscious instructions to "eat this and feel better." We must learn to THINK CONSCIOUSLY of adapting to unpleasant situations in a constructive rather than a self-destructive manner.

For most of us, changing our lifestyle adaptive patterns means learning new things to say to ourselves. Instead of saying "I'll show you" when we're angry, and then sitting on our anger and stuffing our faces, we need to say, "I'm darned angry with this situation, and you and I are going to discuss this." It's easier to change your attitudes than you might think. All you need to do is to BECOME AWARE that you are angry. Hear your voice rise in pitch. Feel your blood pulsate in your head. Experience your stomach tightening up. Know that your hands tend to clench in anger. Take note that your eyes narrow when you are angry. You may even feel the hairs on the back of your neck stand up. These are physiological signals that your body sends you through your nervous system, and they need an appropriate response.

THE DEPRIVATION-REWARD CYCLE

I have observed many obese people. When they are "dieting" intensively and dropping weight rapidly, they have a will of steel that would challenge any warrior's. But once they reach their desired weight, they seem driven to eat like crazy. Many of them describe this "newly thin, driven to eat" state as a time of indiscriminate bingeing. They will eat cold mashed potatoes, leftover soggy fries — *anything* that fills them up. Interestingly enough, once these people return to their "normal" obese state — one which, in the past, they maintained for a long period of time — they become selective about their food again. No longer will last night's sticky spaghetti suffice. Now they are more picky. Now they'll walk a mile through snow, sleet, and hail to get their "fix" of Snickers bars. Sound familiar?

One woman comes to my mind as an example of this vicious deprivation-reward cycle of dieting. I'll call her Vickie. When I met her, Vickie had gone through a six-year cycle of dieting and regaining. At age fifteen, she had weighed 120 pounds. Then she started to gain, and within a year she was up to 165 pounds. By age seventeen, she was back down to 120 pounds. When she graduated from high school a year later, she weighed 165 pounds. This cycle repeated itself again and again. Finally, she came into private therapy with me.

We discussed how she felt when she got back to 120 pounds.

She said she felt emotionally "high" and excited about life — and ENORMOUSLY HUNGRY. She could not resist any food she saw. She told me that her *body* seemed to urge her to return to 165 pounds. The first time she reached 120 pounds, she fought with herself every day to stop her indiscriminate bingeing, but to no avail. When she approached 160 pounds, however, she noticed that she no longer ate everything in sight. She still binged, but much more selectively. Once back at her full 165 pounds, she leveled off to her "normal" pattern of bingeing on selected foods.

Vickie was terribly discouraged when we met. So we began the process of unraveling some of the subconscious messages from her childhood — what I call "mental tapes" — and we found some good ones. She had, for example, one very strong conditioning tape that said, "Live for today, for tomorrow may never come." Another tape told her to "eat it while you have it."

Where did Vickie get these tapes? She came from a poor Southern family, and life was almost literally "feast or famine." When the crops came in, they ate well. But during the winter all they had were their canned or dried foods, and they had to make them last. Vickie told me that when she was a child she dreaded the cold weather and its promise of only one meal a day. Even as an adult she could not bear cold weather, and would wear sweaters or coats when others did not need them.

What seemed to be happening with Vickie, as with many overweight people, was a combination of early childhood conditioning, which prompted her to "eat while you can," and a physiological "set point," which pushed her to fill up her fat cells again. According to set-point theory, the weight regulatory mechanism (WRM), located in the hypothalamus of the brain, triggers the body either to waste or to conserve energy in order to maintain the body's set-point weight — much as the body's temperature-regulating system causes shivering in the cold or sweating in the heat to maintain the body's optimal temperature. When a person tries to lower her weight by dieting, the body responds by decreasing the metabolic rate so that fewer calories are used. At the same time, the body increases appetite to ensure adequate caloric intake. Thus, for those whose set points, through years of overeating, have settled at an obese level, the brain and body "conspire" to maintain their body weights at an unhealthy, high level.

Vickie and I determined that she was probably responding to food on both an emotional and a physiological level. Emotionally (subconsciously), she was afraid to run out of food. Physiologically, she was driven to fill up those fat cells to return to her familiar set point of 165 pounds. Of course this was hardly good news to Vickie. Not only did her emotional self prompt her to eat while she had the chance, her physiological self was also pushing her to get back to her comfortable, "safe" set point of 165 pounds. How could she get out of this bind? She felt doomed.

I'm sure that many of you reading this can identify with Vickie. Well, you will be thrilled to learn that she did find a way out, and she has maintained a weight of 127 pounds (a more realistic weight for her) for nearly four years.

How did she do it? How can you do it, too?

It was much simpler than Vickie could imagine. Our first step was to acknowledge that there was a part of her subconscious mind that was fearful of the long, cold, foodless winter. She began doing a Reflective Relearning technique for ten minutes every day. She got herself to a quiet, isolated spot and repeated to herself that she had ample food for as long as she needed it. This was Phase One of our plan. In the second part of this book, you will learn specific ways of doing the Reflective Relearning process yourself.

Like most of us, Vickie started out a "doubting Thomas." She told me frankly that she would try the ten-minute technique because it was a last resort for her, but she didn't think that just talking to her subconscious mind would work. In fact, she was so embarrassed about doing the procedure that she refused to tell people, for fear that they would think she was crazy or dabbling in the occult or who knows what!

She promised, however, that she would do the entire process faithfully for six weeks, for ten minutes a day. Meanwhile, she also began following a sensible dietary plan to allow her body to move toward a lower weight. Of course, like the true-blue dieter she was, she did great. For several weeks, she never swerved off the path.

As Vickie approached 140 pounds, she and I began Phase Two. This was to begin to allow her subconscious mind to work not only on the emotional aspect of her weight but also on the physiological mechanism, the set point. You see, today we know that such physiological phenomena as the set point are to some degree under conscious control. There was a time when people thought that these responses were automatic. Today, because of research with biofeedback machines, we know that many of these "automatic physiological states" may fall under conscious control when the individual learns to focus attention in these areas.

To do this new work, Vickie added ten minutes to her Reflective Relearning schedule. Now she was spending twenty minutes a day with herself, telling her subconscious mind and her body that she had no need to fill up her fat cells. She repeated an affirmation over and over to herself, hundreds of times, that she would fill her life with other delights, but she would not fill up her fat cells. She still felt a bit ridiculous sitting alone in her bedroom every day making affirmation after affirmation, and she was, reasonably, still afraid to reach her goal-weight for the same reason she had always feared getting there — that she might rapidly regain her weight.

Vickie was seeing me once a week now, and we would review how she was doing on her Reflective Relearning. She was growing more used to it and even looked forward to her "self-time," but she confessed that she still didn't really think it was going to work. I told her to STOP THINKING AND START DOING! This is called the "Do-Do" principle: *Do* do it! Vickie would agree, and off she would go until the next week. Finally, she got close to her goal. She was now at 126 pounds, and she was frightened. I assured her over and over that she had invested many hundreds of minutes of preventive measures against the old drive to get back to 165. Her investment would stand her in good stead. The day she got to 120, she called me in a panic. Again, I reassured her. She scheduled an appointment for the next day.

When Vickie arrived at my office, she was calmer than I had ever seen her. Beaming, she said that she knew it had been only one day since she had obtained her weight goal, but she felt no immediate need to binge — and she considered that in itself to be a miracle. It may have been a miracle, but she also needed to take credit for all the preventive work she had done to ensure that once she obtained her desired weight, she would keep it. Now she wouldn't think of returning to her old weight.

As a result of her determination and the counseling she had received, Vickie not only gained her desired weight but also gained insight into her blocks against doing regular exercise. She had also begun a supplemental weight control program to help her monitor her daily eating patterns and know exactly how many calories she was taking in. Her daily Reflective Relearning sessions were now helping her to "get her shift together" — to make the all-important transition from obtaining to *maintaining* her desired weight.

Vickie used a combination of techniques — including healthy eating patterns and regular exercise — to obtain and maintain her desired weight. Yet she feels that the time she spent (and still spends) doing her Reflective Relearning was the key to changing her lifestyle adaptive patterns.

Vickie is still somewhat amazed that she has had no desire to binge. She can't figure it out logically. But that's no surprise: The right brain and the subconscious mind know nothing about logic or rational thinking. Yet they have an intuitive wisdom of their own, which you can use if you choose to do so. Constructive change through Reflective Relearning isn't as hard as most people think. Once we make up our minds to sit quietly for ten minutes a day to reprogram our behavior, the rest is history. Our subconscious minds and right brains do what they do best — they come up with the "how to" in an illogical, irrational, unreasonable manner. Nevertheless, they are powerful mechanisms, and all I can do is encourage you to use them, as I encouraged Vickie.

As scientists discover more and more evidence that our "unconscious" bodily processes are subject to conscious control, an increasing number of people are learning techniques that allow them to change what was once thought to be automatic, uncontrollable behavior. Yes, perhaps heredity has programmed you to fill up your fat cells, but what we are learning about the right brain and the subconscious mind shows that you can countermand this drive to eat.

You can't do it solely with your logical, left brain — at least not if you want to change your eating patterns for "good." Like Vickie, you must work on FAITH, which expands beyond belief. I once heard that the word "decision" literally means "to cut away from." Vickie made a decision. She cut away from her left-brain denial that reprogramming her right brain and subconscious mind could change her, permanently. And for nearly four years she has reaped the rewards. So can you.

By the way, Vickie still does her daily ten minutes of Reflective Relearning — although not for her desired weight. She has that, and her new subconscious orientation to food usually makes it effortless for her to maintain it. Now she works on seeing herself moving ahead in her career. She told me not long ago, when we met socially, that her career is really getting in line now. Next she will be working on getting a special man into her life. Watch out for Vickie: there's no stopping her now!

SOME FACTS ABOUT YOUR FIGURE

You can see that there are other ways to get around barriers than running into them over and over again. You can jump over the barrier, or go around it, or you can even tunnel underneath it. There are ways to get around the facts about fat which will allow your figure to be the way you wish it to be.

Let's start by looking at the definitions of some terms we need to use when we are discussing eating behaviors:

Hunger: A compelling physical need for food, sometimes accompanied by a painful sensation or state of weakness. Hunger pangs are somewhat controlled by the level of glucose in the blood.

Appetite: Desire for a specific food. Often confused with hunger, appetite is less physiological and more related to mental and emotional drives. Appetite is related to memories of good meals (and probably also the good company and pleasant times). With continued deprivation, appetite becomes hunger.

Obesity: Accumulation of excess fat. People are deemed **clinically obese** when they are twenty percent or more over their standard weight as suggested by the actuarial chart, which lists medically approved healthy weights for men, women, and children based on height, sex, age, and size of frame. These actuarial charts are based on the mortality figures of life insurance policy-holders. **Morbid obesity** is the condition of being two or more times over the weight suggested by the actuarial chart. In doctor talk, "morbid" means "diseased." Individuals who are morbidly obese run a high risk of serious illness or death. Yet even those who are only ten percent above their normal weight may experience serious health risks.

While obesity may occasionally be caused by glandular disorders, in the vast majority of cases obesity is caused by overeating and underexercising. Obese individuals oxidize glucose at a lower metabolic rate.

Obesity is measured by skinfold tests (using calipers) at four body sites: at the biceps and triceps (arm muscles), at the lower-middle spine, and under the collar bone. If you can "pinch an inch" in any of these areas, keep reading!

Obesity can also be measured by the water displacement test, an excellent test that tells you the percentage of fatty tissue in your body. This is not an easy test to do on yourself, but it is administered at many hospitals, at some university medical centers, and some YMCAs or health clubs. Some of these places offer this test as a community service during certain times of the year. Call your nearest university for information.

Desirable Weight: The height-to-weight guidelines given in the actuarial charts help to give an idea of what a person's "desirable" or healthy weight is. However, these charts do not consider many factors that are important when trying to draw the line between desirable weight and overweight for any individual, factors like age, family history, racial origin, even occupation. In their 1985 report the National Institutes of Health (NIH) suggest using another measurement called the **Body Mass Index.** To figure out your body mass index you simply divide your weight in kilograms by the square of your height in meters (no need to be alarmed, just get out your calculator and use the formula below!):

To get kilograms, divide your weight in pounds by 2.2: _____ (A)

To get meters, divide your height in inches by 39.4: _____ (B)

Now, square B, *i.e.* B x B = _____ (B^2)

Divide A by B^2. A/B^2 = Body Mass Index = _____

Example:

A weight of 160 pounds = $\dfrac{160}{2.2}$ kilograms = 72.5 kilograms (A)

A height of 5 ft. 3 inches = $\dfrac{63}{39.4}$ meters = 1.6 meters (B)

B × B = 2.56 (B^2), and
A/B^2 = Body Mass Index (BMI) = 28.3

The higher the body mass, the more serious the overweight problem. A desirable body mass range for men is from 22 to 24, above 28.5 is overweight, and a body mass above 33 has serious health implications. For women the desirable range is 21 to 23, above 27.5 is overweight, and a body mass above 31.5 should be a danger signal.

Remember, it is a *fact* (at least a medically accepted fact) that high caloric intake during the first few months of life may lead to an increase in the number of fat cells in the body. This can predispose the child to obesity later in life. After the first few months of life, the number of fat cells we possess remains constant — what varies is whether the fat cells are "full" (grapes) or "empty" (raisins). Warning: Don't think that a plump baby is cute — put him on an appropriate eating program!

Another psychologically accepted fact is that obese people (unlike nonobese people) don't necessarily feel hungry when they get appropriate physiological cues, such as stomach contractions and low blood sugar levels. On the other hand, fat people may respond to inappropriate stimuli with what they think are feelings of hunger. For example, a fat person may eat simply because the hands of the clock are pointing to "dinner-time." There is also evidence that a fat person eats because he was conditioned as a child to eat when his emotions ran high (adrenaline can trigger eating). Studies indicate that anxiety and stress decrease eating tendencies in lean people but increase them in fat people.

There have been several psychological studies of eating-by-the-clock behavior. In one clever study, for example, the researcher fixed the clocks to go slow or fast. When people responded to the time the inaccurate clock showed, rather than to the actual time, there were some interesting results. The great majority of over-weight people in the study ate before their mealtime, when the clock was set to go fast. In one instance, the researcher left a box of crackers and some cheese lying about, with the directions, "Help yourself." Most of the overweight people, thinking that it was past their mealtime, did help themselves. The majority of the slim people, however, did not. When the experiment was over, the overweight people were questioned about why they had eaten. Were they hungry, bored, or what? The majority of those who had eaten responded that they had felt hungry — and besides, it was already past their usual dinnertime. In reality, they had eaten one hour earlier than their usual mealtime, because they had been watching a fast clock. The thinner people reported that they had not eaten because they had not wanted to spoil their dinner.

THE DECEPTIVE Ds:
DIETS, DRUGS, AND DISSECTION

As we can see, the facts behind fat are emotional as well as physiological. Fat people think differently from thin people. Those of us who are fat may be able to obtain our desired weight through iron will and self-deprivation, but unless we learn to think differently about food and eating, we haven't a chance when it comes to maintaining and sustaining our desired weight.

Let me show you what I mean with a look at some of the

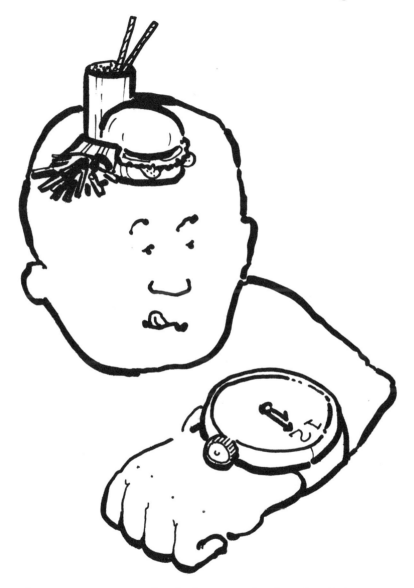

A person may eat simply because the hands of the clock
are pointing to "dinner-time."

old, traditional ways of *losing* weight. In the past, the scientific community, including medical professionals, believed that certain bodily responses were beyond conscious control. Obese patients were treated as though they needed a great deal of external control to fend off obesity. Many doctors and most of their patients believed that they needed something outside themselves in order to control their "automatic," compulsive eating patterns.

The Diet Dilemma

For many of us, that "something outside" ourselves has been a DIET — that hateful disciplinarian with which we do battle year in and year out (usually right after the holidays, or two weeks before that special event). If we are wise, we go to the doctor; if we aren't so wise, we pick up the latest fad diet book and get a diet. We then go on this diet, no matter how horrible or severe it might be, for a given length of time to reach a specific weight goal. We tell ourselves that we'll stay on this doggone diet no matter what until we reach that magic number on the scales.

The subconscious mind agrees that you are going on that special "bees knees and poached gnat" diet until you get to 120 pounds, or you'll die in the attempt. Okay, fine, now you're there. Now what? Most people who deprive themselves of foods they like are subconsciously anxious to get out of the deprivational mode and into its counterpart. And what is always the counterpart to deprivation? Yep! We go out and reward ourselves because we have been so good. Of course, most of us have not thought past our noses to just how we will reward ourselves, so we quickly slide back toward the refrigerator, where we've always found instant rewards. After all, the subconscious part of us remembers how good eating made us feel in the past. Why pass up a surefire, tried-and-true way of feeling better?

This is the real tragedy of dieting. Many people admit that each new fad diet leaves them fatter than before! Each time, they get more remorseful and more depressed for having "failed" again, and the weight comes back on quicker than it came off.

There is a diet for every letter of the alphabet, starting with

"A" for the Atkins diet, "B" for the Beverly Hills diet, "C" for the Cambridge diet, "D" for the Drinking Man's diet, "E" for Eating is OK — and the list goes on. Not all of these diets are poorly constructed; many of them are nutritionally sound. What's wrong is that they don't go far enough. Almost all diets focus on getting you to your desired weight. Great. Who hasn't been there, at least once in a lifetime? But when it comes to keeping you at your desired weight, diets are no help. Whenever you and I go on a temporary diet (which is what they almost always are), we focus on a temporary weight loss, and the devil take the hindmost as far as what will happen after we reach our weight goal. It is almost as though we are too burdened with the dieting process itself to bother with the thought of what comes next. Most people are so intent upon their diets that they truly have no energy to focus on the lifestyle changes they desperately need to make if they are to KEEP their desired weight.

This left-brain approach to weight has prevailed in our culture far too long. Some pioneers in the field of weight control have attempted to reach beyond these shortsighted plans: Weight Watchers, Overeaters Anonymous, and TOPS, for example. They have recognized the value of follow-through and group support for overweight people, both while they are on the dietary program and after they have reached their desired weight. Such organizations realize the importance of the emotional aspects of eating and do not attempt to take the purely intellectual approach of telling people to stick to their diets and everything will be fine.

The Perils Of Pills And Potions

Okay, so diets don't work. Where to turn next? Well, if you want to stick with the old left-brain "external control" school, you might try pills.

Looking back over the past twenty-five or thirty years, we see the rise in popularity of the diet pill. The magic pill! The pill that can kill any appetite! The glorious pill that causes fat to fall from my bones while I sit passively, or even enjoy myself. Pop one of these miracle drugs and watch the fat just melt off your body!

It wasn't too long ago that a lot of people believed in pills as the cure-all for obesity. Accompanying the old-fashioned belief that being fat was beyond a person's control was the belief that a person needs to be "sick" in order to become thin. Some people would actually make themselves physically ill in order to get pills to make them thin — and thus well again. Once more, the idea was that the cure lay somewhere outside the power of the individual. Overweight people simply saw their doctors to get a prescription for a diet pill and then sat back to await magical, instant thinness.

And boy, these were some pills! Amphetamines ("uppers" or "speed"), and adrenergic drugs to suppress appetite. Metabolic medications to rev up our body engines and make them burn more calories. Diuretics to help us shed water weight for an illusion of quick weight loss. Laxatives to speed food through the digestive system before it could turn to fat — or nourish our bodies.

The only problem was, these pills had their side effects: nervousness, irritability, insomnia, dry mouth, diarrhea, blurred vision, dizziness, high blood pressure, dehydration, damage to our physical organs, physical addiction — you name it. Even some of the nonprescription products for weight control — the diet "candies," starch blockers, and liquid diets — could cause everything from nausea to kidney damage. And, being easily accessible, they were also easy to abuse. Of course, the side effects weren't the only problem. As with diets, people found themselves back on the same old loss-gain teeter-totter. All those side effects for nothing!

Placing our hopes in such "cures" is again a case of the patient playing a passive role in his health, trusting the physician to dispense the pills and control the situation. This old paradigm of passive patient and omnipotent doctor is yielding to a new model of self-responsibility. Prescriptions for pills and potions to control weight are still made, but not to the extent they were in the past. With the vast documentation on the side effects of diet pills, many physicians are much more cautious about prescribing these "miracle" drugs. And patients themselves are becoming more choosy about which prescriptions they take, and whether to use diet drugs at all.

Surgical Interventions

In cases of extreme obesity, surgical procedures have been used to assist individuals in getting to their desired weight. These procedures include intestinal bypass surgery, gastric surgery (stomach stapling), and jaw-wiring.

Such procedures are not magic cures either. There is high risk of side effects, and unpleasant or even life-threatening consequences if the patient fails to make significant changes in his lifestyle and eating patterns. Again, the notion that "something out there" will take care of your weight challenge for you, while you blissfully continue in your old habits, is a myth when it comes to these surgical procedures.

As proof of this, let's take a look at what happens in intestinal bypass surgery. Put quite simply, the surgeon re-routes the passage from the stomach to the large intestine, bypassing much of the small intestine. The theory is that if food is in the body for less time, the body will absorb fewer calories.

Candidates for this type of surgery must usually be at least 100 pounds over their actuarial chart body weight and must go through rigorous psychological screening to determine whether this "last-ditch" method of intervention is indeed necessary. Furthermore, physicians warn anyone who chooses this surgery of the significant risks and consequences of the procedure. There is often a misconception that after the operation the patient can eat anything he likes, whenever he likes, and stay thin. This is simply not so. Intestinal bypass patients may only eat from a highly restricted list of foods *for the rest of their lives* after the operation. Otherwise they face the consequences: painful, foul-smelling gas; frequent bowel movements; diarrhea; and the emotional complications that accompany these problems. There are also serious risks during the operation: pneumonia, clotting of the blood, and a five percent mortality rate.

All of these complications must be fully recognized by anyone seriously considering surgery for obesity. There are cases in which surgery is justified and even necessary, but only when the patient is willing to commit to major lifestyle changes.

I recall the first time that I counseled a patient — we'll call him Joe — who was considering intestinal bypass surgery. When I met him, Joe weighed 643 pounds. He was just over six feet tall and had a sixty-five inch waist. Obese since childhood and never able to recall feeling like he had a normal body, Joe had begun dieting when he was six years old, and dieting had been a major part of his life for the past thirty-four years.

When we began counseling, Joe's job was in grave jeopardy, as it entailed traveling by plane and meeting new people. He had to purchase two airline tickets (for two seats, because one wasn't wide enough), board early, and deplane last. He also found that he could not walk from the plane to the baggage pickup without becoming so winded that he had to sit and rest every half-dozen steps. His employers had reluctantly told him that he had to reduce his weight within the next three months or be terminated. He was a high producer for his company and they sincerely wanted him to continue, yet they felt they could no longer put him through such living hell on business trips. While at the plant Joe got around with relative ease, because he rode a cart, walked slowly, and paced himself. But traveling was a different story.

I learned that Joe had done just about everything he could think of to reach a "normal" weight, but each attempt had left him only more frustrated and angry, which, of course, had led to further eating binges. He now felt that unless he shed some weight quickly, he might as well be dead.

I reviewed the case with the surgeon, and we both decided to ask Joe to consider a modified medical fast for at least two months and then to reconsider the surgery. Joe reluctantly agreed to do this. Yet, after only three and a half weeks, he was back in the doctor's office. He had lost a grand total of one and a half pounds. He simply could not or would not stay on the medical fast. He was full of anguish and self-hatred for having "failed again."

At this point, the surgeon decided to consider the surgery, as Joe's blood pressure was surely going to cause an early death if his depression didn't. He therefore asked Joe to follow the recommended format, which requires a patient to seek the counsel of other medical doctors using alternative procedures to make sure that he had chosen the right one.

Joe returned a week later. He had talked to two other physicians and had reviewed their particular surgical procedures. Joe knew that stomach stapling would not work, because he knew himself well enough to know that he would continue eating too much. Patients who have their stomachs stapled must eat in small portions, and Joe felt that he could not trust himself to do this. Another procedure he considered also left too many opportunities to "cheat" and still get calories, so Joe decided against it, too. And jaw-wiring wouldn't work — he could drink malts!

Waiting for the surgery, Joe experienced great anxiety, fearing that at the last minute he might not qualify. Finally, after several sessions with the surgeon and me, Joe felt ready both psychologically and physically to face the operation.

The surgery went well. There were few complications, and Joe recovered rapidly. He soon began to drop weight. Like all patients who undergo surgery for weight reduction, he now had to relearn all of his eating habits or suffer the severe physical consequences — gaseous and abdominal pain.

The last time I saw Joe, his blood pressure was near normal and, after many months, his weight was nearing normal. He suffered the common side effects, such as gas and diarrhea, when he did not eat appropriately, but as long as he ate right and followed the doctor's orders, he did relatively well.

If you are considering surgery for obesity, be sure you select a doctor who knows of the latest procedures and their side effects. Discuss your thoughts with your family, and make sure they approve, or at least understand why you are having this surgery. Ask to talk to previous patients to see how they feel. And above all, be prepared for the fact that you will be making major changes not only in your eating patterns but in other areas of your life as well. Like diets, surgery cannot work unless you are prepared to change your entire life.

THE NEW WAY

As our new age moves forward, we are seeing more and more evidence that the older, traditional methods of "losing" weight —

methods in which we relinquish control to our medical prac-
titioners and expect them to do our work for us — no longer fit
with the general trend toward self-responsibility for health. More
and more, we see people making sophisticated choices about their
health care, with their doctors as guides, not gods. It is in keeping
with this new principle of self-responsibility that greater numbers
of people are looking beyond the immediate goal of obtaining
their desired weight to lifestyle changes that will also allow them
to maintain and sustain that weight.

Another aspect of this trend toward self-directedness is the
growing interest in learning to reprogram behavior through our
most powerful tool — the mind. There is an increasing gravitation
toward "naturalness" in all phases of life, from eating foods with
fewer additives to giving birth without anesthesia. All these trends
point in the same direction: toward a greater self-reliance, and less
passive dependence on someone or something external to
"cure" us.

People are learning to reprogram themselves through classes in
relaxation, meditation, and self-hypnosis. If you are one of the
many people interested in learning how to make use of internal,
rather than external controls, you will find much more about this
process in subsequent chapters. Through Reflective Relearning,
you can learn to obtain, maintain, and sustain your desired weight
for life — with you at the helm, directing the process and getting
what you want.

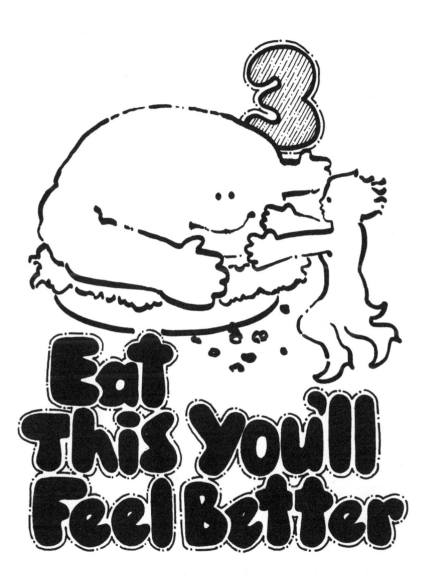

3

Eat This You'll Feel Better

Dear Fat,

You've protected me from new and scary adventures. You've kept me safe and at a distance. You've been with me throughout my life, providing me with excuses not to do things I don't want to do, and even things I want to do — things that frighten me. You've been my scapegoat. But now I'm tired of you, fat! I don't need you any longer. Filling full is not fulfilling my needs; you're not helping me to be happy. I don't need your wall of security anymore. Why did I ever think I needed you, anyway? So long, fat!

IN MY YEARS OF WORKING WITH OVERWEIGHT PEOPLE, I have learned that the first step we need to take to obtain, maintain, and sustain our desired weight is to recognize that weight is a product of our emotions and the thinking patterns connected with those emotions. To do that, we need to make our logical, "conscious" left brain aware of the pictorial, "automatic" images through which our right brain connects our emotions with food. Writing a letter to our fat, as trivial or contrived as it may first appear, is one of the most effective exercises I have found for taking that first step.

The letter that opens this chapter is one example from my thick file of "Dear Fat" letters — letters written by formerly fat people who took that first step of understanding why they thought they needed to be fat. This letter, however, is particularly appropriate because it asks, "Why did I ever *think* I needed you?" In the next two chapters, we will explore why we "think" we need our fat, and just how the functioning of the right brain plays into that thinking.

The use of quotation marks around "think" is deliberate, because the thought process that leads us to overeat usually isn't deliberate. Instead, it is often a subconscious thought process — and there's the catch! It is difficult, if not impossible, to change behavior that is triggered by subconscious, right-brain-influenced thoughts unless we first move those thoughts to the left-brain realm of consciousness. Writing a "Dear Fat" letter is one way of doing just that. We begin to see our inner relationship with fat and gain insight into how we allowed ourselves to gain the unwanted weight in the first place.

THOUGHT → ACTION → FORM

The first thing that we need to understand, then, is that *weight is in consciousness.* What? What does that mean?

Let's start with basics. The direction of the world is from thought to action to form. That is, first someone has a *thought* (a conception, a beginning). That thought provokes *action* (behavior). The result, or outcome, is a *form.* For instance, I had an idea (a thought) to write this book. Next, I took action, I sat down and wrote a rough draft of the ideas I wanted to present. Now, many months and many drafts later, you are holding the final form — a printed book.

This flow from thought to action to form is a universal law, and it is an essential concept for you to grasp. Only by controlling our *thought* processes — that is, by becoming aware of what we are thinking, recognizing the actions toward which those thoughts could lead, and altering our thoughts accordingly — can we begin to change our behavior. This is where the *action* part comes in. Now we can take the necessary intervening action to bring about the final, desired form. In more familiar terms, we begin consciously to break old habits so as to obtain our desired body weight.

Too many of us, in trying to obtain that desired form, place the cart before the horse. We concentrate first on the final form (the body weight we wish to "lose" to), then we choose a course of action (usually a diet) that we believe will lead to that form, and then we expect our thinking process to conform to that action.

This path is the reverse of what it needs to be. In order to obtain, maintain, and sustain our desired weight, we must begin with our thoughts. It is fruitless to spend hours planning new diets, searching for miracle drugs, or pursuing radical surgical measures. Instead, we must start with ourselves: What's in the back of my mind when I'm eating when I *know* that I'm not physically hungry? What prompts me to return again and again to the refrigerator when I'm alone at night? What's going on in my right brain and subconscious mind when I find myself eating to "show" somebody something? When I "swallow my anger," what is the unexpressed anger I'm swallowing? How is it that I seem to eat automatically the moment I feel frustrated or under pressure at work? What, in other words, is at the root of my eating patterns?

Thinking is the proper starting point — the only starting point — if we wish to succeed. Focusing on the feelings behind the thoughts behind the actions behind the form is the only way to begin to make a lasting change in that final form. Mother Nature works this way: There's a thought, then an action, then a form.

To get to the right form, then, we must invest some time learning about our thought patterns. It is amazing how many hundreds of thoughts — right-brain and left-brain, subconscious and conscious — can pass through our minds in a very short time, and almost at the same time. We need to allow ourselves time to learn to sort out and become aware of these thoughts. Later on in this book, specific, step-by-step methods of becoming aware are presented. For the moment, however, let's take a look at how the thought-action-form principle applies to body weight.

WHEN WAS THE LAST TIME YOU WERE FORCE-FED?

After years of working with people who are overweight, I have concluded that, for most of us, being fat (having an undesired form) is the result of faulty problem solving (faulty action), which, in turn, is the result of faulty thinking. That is, we have an emotion which may not be fully conscious, one that leads us to a tension-reducing behavior. Because we have learned to reduce tension with food, we turn to eating as a way of "solving" our problems. As we shall see later, this faulty problem solving is directly connected with early childhood learning patterns surrounding food.

We have already established that we must learn to change our thinking patterns in order to change our bodies. This means that we must learn to accept that, for many of us, overeating is a choice. Thus, in a roundabout way, *being fat is a choice.* Needless to say, many people rebel at this idea. I hope you have not thrown this book into the fireplace!

Let's back up a second and see how this works. Rarely does a person start the day by thinking, "Today, I'll set out to see how much I can eat, so as to become fat." It doesn't work that directly. On the contrary, many overweight people begin each day with a great promise to themselves that they are going to be good and stick to their diets. When, by the end of the day, they have slipped back into the old pattern of overeating, they would hardly consider their behavior something they had planned to do. "I really wanted to stick with it," they might say to themselves, "but things are so crazy at work right now, I just had to do something to calm down." The "choice," according to this way of thinking, was to stick to the diet, but that choice was foiled by external forces.

To expose the faultiness of this kind of thinking, I often ask groups of overweight people that if they don't think that being fat is a choice, when was the last time they were tied to a chair and forcefed? During one group session, when we were exploring this idea, one of the women in the group became really tickled, and she started laughing uproariously, causing the rest of us to laugh along with her. Finally, she said, "Fantasy of fantasies — imagine being tied to a chair and forcefed!" This woman had been on a modified fasting program for many months. All she had eaten for days was a liquid dietary supplement, and to her the idea of being forcefed was delightful. It was something that at least a part of her would have liked to have happen — something that she might *choose* for herself. We all got a laugh out of that! We also gained insight into some of the "forces" that lead to fat. Those forces are internal, not external — the thoughts that lead to action and result in the form of our bodies.

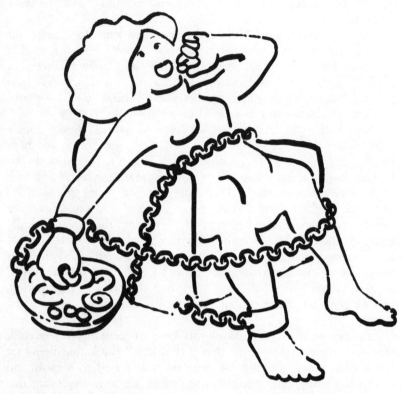

I often ask people that if they don't think being fat is a choice, when were they last tied to a chair and force fed?

YOUR RIGHT BRAIN: TEAM PLAYER OR CO-CONSPIRATOR?

Let's relate this process directly to food. I have a thought, such as "I'm hungry." I take action: I explore the refrigerator; I eat. I end up with a new form: My body weight changes. Of course, when life is moving along in a nice, orderly, uncomplicated manner — when I really am viscerally hungry — this process works wonderfully. The Catch-22 comes when I complicate the process. I say, "I *think* I'm hungry," when actually what I am is angry, bored, frustrated, or whatever. My faulty thinking starts a chain of faulty actions, and I eat rather than express my anger, go to a movie, take a walk, or otherwise deal directly with my feelings. I'm not physically hungry. I just *think* I'm hungry because I am experiencing some emotion which prompts behavior. This behavior may well be to reach for food, which I have associated with reducing tension.

I have chained my emotions to food. Many of us do that. We have learned to substitute the subconscious, right-brain thought of food for conscious, left-brain thinking ("What do I *really* want?"). Over the years, we have learned by means of many subtle suggestions — an arched eyebrow, a look of disappointment, a loving hug, and so on — that we must eat something for approval, for comfort, or for love. These subtle cues, which have occurred in proximity to food and eating, are faithfully recorded in the right brain and relegated to the subconscious mind. This is how we have learned to eat in order to feel better, no matter what the problem is.

HOW WE BECOME FAT: CHILDHOOD TAPES

How did our emotionally charged right brain learn this head-in-the-sand, one-size-fits-all approach to solving our problems? After all, no one consciously believes that eating a half-gallon of ice cream will appease the boss or prevent nuclear war. How did our right-brain, emotional side learn to cue us to reach for food when we feel unrest or frustration or some other uncomfortable emotion?

These associational patterns were set when we were infants. When you and I were very small, we experienced hunger pangs. All we could do to express our needs before we could talk was to cry. And when we cried, relief was on the way. Mommy, or someone close to us, came along and offered a bottle or, if we were lucky, a warm breast. Not only were we sated with food, but we were also held while we were being fed — held nice and close to Mommy's body. We were held and fed and burped. And, if we were parented well, we usually got coos, pats, rubs on the back, and kisses along with our food. This association of food with love and security was drilled into our pictorial, emotional right-brain memories and our subconscious minds daily, for months and months. We got hungry, we cried, we got food and love and reassurance, and we went to sleep. A nice life if you can get it!

As we got older, these associations were reinforced. One way we learned to eat when we were bored or angry or had a skinned knee or couldn't have that electric train set was when Mom said, "Here, eat this. You'll feel better." And do you know what? We did feel better! There's the rub. We actually did feel better once we ate the food. And the emotion that was disturbing us was temporarily laid to rest. We heard our mothers telling us to "eat this and feel better" over and over, day after day. Remember, the subconscious mind, unlike the critical conscious mind, does not make value judgments about what it is told. Repeated ideas are accepted by and stored in the subconscious — especially when we are little kids and our relatively immature left brains are less apt to respond with a judgmental, "Now wait a minute!" Likewise, the right brain picks up the connection between hurt (skinned knee) and food ("Eat this, you'll feel better") and, after many such experiences, learns to produce a *gestalt* — a holistic mental response to new situations that combines the feelings, thoughts, visual images, and everything else connected with similar situations in the past.

Like the subconscious mind, the right brain simply responds to outside stimuli and the emotions they produce. And it responds nonevaluatively and noncritically. The right brain produces, all at once, the "big picture" composed of every emotion, eyebrow arch, sensation of pain, smell of cinnamon, and other memory trace associated with the situation at hand. Then it communicates this picture to the left brain, which is prompted to take action on the basis of the past behaviors. In essence, the subconscious mind and the right brian say to the conscious mind and left brain: "Okay, here's what we got in our files (memory traces) for such situations. And here's what you normally do in such situations."

I have a term for these habituated right-brain and subconscious patterns: *mental tapes*. When we run up against a situation that creates uncomfortable emotions, a button is pressed in the right brain and subconscious mind, and a tape begins to play. Unless our left brain becomes consciously aware of these tapes, we tend, like automatons, to follow their commands.

Let's examine some of the childhood tapes that have been playing over and over in our right brains, triggering subconscious memories that translate into faulty behavior. How many of these do you recognize?

> "Clean your plate. Remember all of those starving children in
> _____." (Fill in the blank.)

Some of us got the tape about the starving children in China. How about India? Africa? I was told about the starving Armenians. Now bear in mind that, like you, I was merely a small child. I had no concept of "Armenian." And since I didn't have the foggiest notion of what an Armenian was, I did the logical thing. My immature right brain made a loose association and came up with the closest image it could link with the verbal prompt "Armenian" — armadillo. So there I sat in Eldon, Missouri, staring at the peas on my plate, my right brain picturing all those armadillos lying around with their stiff little legs up in the air. Armadillos that I had personally killed because I wouldn't eat my peas.

Here are some more tapes that many of us picked up as children:

> "Don't cry. Look, here's a cookie (or lollipop or ice cream cone). Now isn't that better?"

> "If you eat everything on your plate, you can have some dessert." (Sure. Great. Now we are reinforced with white sugar for eating more than we needed or desired — sugar to make us nice and hyperactive.)

> "I baked this JUST FOR YOU. How can you possibly turn down Grandma's fresh apple pie? And here's some yummy ice cream to go on top. I know you just love it when it's all

melted like that."

"Open wide! Here comes the airplane flying food into your open hanger. Look! It's just crammed full of goodies to make you nice and strong."

"Come on, now. Just three more spoonfuls and you're all through. Tell you what — just two more bites and we'll give the last one to the birdies."

"You're going to sit right there until every last bite is gone, young lady (young man)!"

"Waste not, want not." My parents were products of the Great Depression. So, perhaps, were yours. Therefore, not only was I mandated to waste not, want not, but I got the double whammy. Coupled with "Eat everything in front of you" was "and be grateful!" My father used to say to me, "When I was your age, young lady, I would have given my eyeteeth to have the meal your mother just prepared for you. Now stop talking and start eating." A companion to this "grateful tape" was the "proud tape." It went something like this: "We may not be the wealthiest people on the block, but by golly, we can afford to eat good." When adults grow up knowing what it's like not to have enough food, or at least enough "good stuff" to eat, they are likely to urge their children to "eat everything — and be grateful."

Many of us grew up in that situation, and we are still enacting its mandate and feeling guilty as heck if food is wasted. We keep the smallest bits of leftovers and place them inside little plastic margarine dishes and snap the lid on tight. Where do our leftovers wind up? Correct. At the back of the refrigerator. Once that dab of mashed potatoes has grown its own penicillin, it's okay to throw it away. Otherwise, it's a sin.

WHY WE STAY FAT: ADULT TAPES

Let's speed up this movie to twenty or thirty years later. Now we're not so small. In fact, we may be very, very big. Here we are, our right brains still making the association between love and food, and our subconscious minds prompting us to act on that association.

How do our childhood tapes translate into adult mandates? They're still playing away, of course, but now they've adapted themselves to our adult social roles. For example, whenever friends come to visit, what is one of the first things we do after hanging up their coats? You got it. We ask if they would like a cup of coffee, a drink, or something to snack on. Not to offer food is considered *rude*, and heaven forbid that we be considered rude.

Here are how some of our adult food tapes sound:

"For goodness' sake, eat that little dab of cranberry sauce. What am I supposed to do with a little bit like that? I'll never have room in my fridge for all of these leftovers." (The "waste not, sin not" tape.)

"What? No seconds? I bet I put too much salt in it, huh? Too much sugar? Too spicy? There must be some reason you don't want seconds. You ALWAYS have seconds." (The "Don't you love me?" tape.)

"What do you mean, diet? Not at your own mother's house, you don't. Here, have another piece of your favorite fudgy-wudgy cake. You know I make it only for you. I don't mind that it takes forever — just knowing that my little boy is happy makes it all worthwhile." (The "Prove you love me" tape.)

"It's okay, honey, I like your love handles." (The "Prove you love him (her)" tape.)

"Here, take this leftover pie home with you. Really, I insist. If you leave it here, I'll just eat it." (The "Save me from getting fat" tape — particularly ironic, because it means *you* get fat instead!)

These adult tapes are direct playbacks of our early childhood conditioning about food. We were too small then to resist these suggestions successfully, and we really did think we felt better after eating that cookie for our skinned knee. Why did we think so? Because we were taught so many associations between love and food — some subtle, some obvious. Three of the adult tapes listed above are directly tied to love, and all of them are at least indirectly related to it. Our right brains developed the holistic composite "Food = love = security = fun" — all run together, just like that. This memory trace was stored in the subconscious mind for future use (or misuse).

Half the time when we think we're physically hungry, what we're actually feeling is "head-heart hunger." By this I mean that our emotions prompt us to seek some sort of tension-reducing action, which in turn triggers our right brains to call up an image of what assisted us in the past — food. The subconscious storehouse tells us to eat, and often we do. But what worked well at twenty or thirty months of age may not work as well at twenty or thirty years of age: Now we gain unwanted weight. Old, outmoded emotional associations remain entrenched in our subconscious minds, leading to old, outmoded behaviors. Even though these actions may not serve us to the best advantage, they are familiar, and thus repeated.

As you begin to recognize some of your mental and social tapes about food, however, you become more able to free yourself from them. Remember, there is no change in behavior until we bring these concepts from the subconscious to the conscious level. We must learn to plug substitute tapes into our consciousness — tapes like "I feel lonely; guess I'll take a nice long walk and maybe chat with the neighbors" rather than "I feel lonely; guess I'll eat." When the new suggestion is enacted many times, it becomes as much of a habit as the old one of reaching for food. The key is to form *new* habits through practice.

EXERCISES

1. Take a sheet of paper and draw two vertical lines on it to make three columns. Label the first column "Childhood Tapes."

Label the second "Adult Tapes." Label the third "My Assessment." (See below.)

Childhood Tapes	Adult Tapes	My Assessment
_____	_____	_____
_____	_____	_____
_____	_____	_____

In the first column, list at least five of your childhood tapes
regarding food. Then, for each of these, list a corresponding adult
tape in the second column. (It helps to ask the question, "How
does this childhood tape translate into my adult thinking patterns?" or "How does this childhood tape affect my behavior
today?") In the "Assessment" column, write down your opinion
or evaluation of the message the tape is sending you. Does it
make sense? Does it prompt a wise course of action? Will you be
happy with the outcome of that action? Please DON'T write
down something like "That's a dumb thing to think" — don't put
down an opinion about *yourself*. Simply note how the tapes are
likely to affect your eating patterns and your weight.

2. On a second sheet of paper, draw a vertical line down the
middle to make two columns. Label the first column "Adult
Tapes," and write down your adult tapes from your first sheet of
paper. Label the second column "New Tapes." (See below.)

Adult Tapes	New Tapes
_____	_____
_____	_____
_____	_____

For each old adult tape, list in the second column a new tape
that is based on your assessment of the old tape. For example, if
the old adult tape was "I'd better eat this last spoonful of food,
otherwise it'll go to waste," your assessment might be, "This tape
is invalid; it is keeping me from what I really want — my desired
weight." Now you might chose to write the new tape, "I might as
well toss this last bit; I don't want it now, and it'll be moldy by

the time I'm really hungry again."

3. On a third sheet of paper, write across the top, "If I were at my desired weight...". Make two columns. Label the first "Advantages," the second "Disadvantages."

IF I WERE AT MY DESIRED WEIGHT...

Advantages	Disadvantages

In the first column, list as many pleasurable results as you can of being at your desired weight. In the second column, write down those things that frighten you about being at that weight. Set the list aside for a day or two. Then return to it and rate each advantage and disadvantage on a scale of 1 (not important at all) to 5 (extremely important). Add up the totals for each column.

It is important to remember that persistence pays off. I have talked with many people who thought it would be impossible to shift their thought processes from reaching for food to doing something constructive, yet now they find that they do this habitually, because they have practiced replacing old, destructive tapes with new ones.

You can, too. Don't forget: It took thousands of repetitions to learn to reach for food when you were distressed, so give yourself time to learn to do new things to obtain, maintain, and sustain your desired weight.

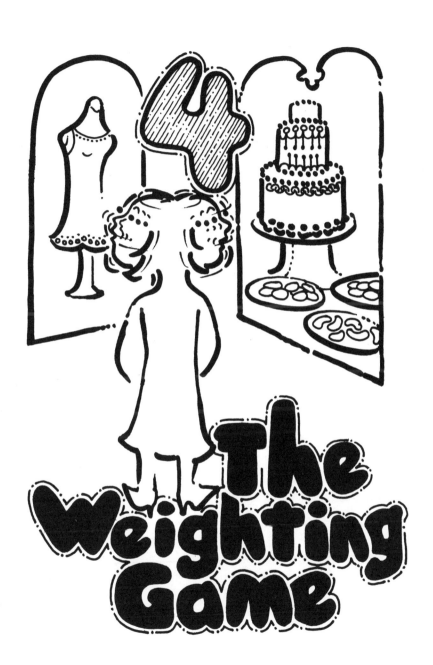

4

The Weighting Game

Dear Fat,

Of all the times to write to you, here it is during the holiday season. It's so hard to resist — everywhere I turn there's food and parties and drinks and more food and more goodies. The first two parties I went to I just sipped a diet cola. I was so good. But I guess the theory about depriving yourself is true — all I know is, suddenly, at the third party, I just went wild. I really pigged out. I am so embarrassed, ashamed, and angry with myself. The worst part is, everyone EXPEC-TED me to pig out. And they were doing it, too — what are parties for? All that free, yummy food! We can always make up for it tomorrow!

And then there's T.V. Talk about a fantasy world! Every other commercial these days is about food and holiday goodies, like if you don't eat them and make them for your family, you're missing out. And you know, I feel like I AM missing out if I can't have those holiday goodies like everyone else! I had my hair done today, and as I thumbed through a magazine, there were dozens of holiday recipes. They made me want to scream!

Guess I'll skip the parties — except for the office party. I told everyone I'm dieting right through New Year's, so I don't dare eat. At Jody and Mike's, they'll expect me to be my regular fat, "jolly" self and chow-down like everyone else.

Wait, I can't believe I'm saying this. I don't really want to miss out on all that fun of being with my friends. Fat, why won't you let me live my life?

SO FAR, WE'VE BEEN DISCUSSING HOW WE GET and keep unwanted fat because of associations that are lodged in our right brain and subconscious. "Erasing" these faulty tapes and replacing them with more appropriate messages would seem to be the ticket to our desired weight. Indeed, this is to a large extent true. The exercises at the end of Chapter 3 are designed to make you aware of the faulty personal tapes that lead to faulty thinking and overeating, and doing them is an important first step.

TAPPING INTO SOCIAL TAPES

There are, however, other tapes that are constantly playing outside our minds, vying for our attention and acceptance. These social tapes are played over the media — television, radio, newspapers, magazines, billboards — and by our families, friends, and co-workers. Social tapes are fresh, external messages that interact with old, internalized associations in the right brain and/or with our intellectual left brain to add to or modify our thoughts and hence our behavior. To the extent that we are "unaware" of them, these messages can influence our behavior via the subconscious mind, without our ever consciously recognizing them, analyzing them, or making a choice to act on them.

Social tapes play an essential role in survival and what psychologists call "socialization" — the process whereby we learn to live with our fellow human beings. As we were growing up, we learned that putting our fingers into a flame would result in pretty painful consequences. If we were unlucky, we learned that lesson the hard way — through direct, painful experience, rather than through a parents' social-tape warning. Likewise, we learned that a red traffic light means "stop"; that hitting our kid sister when she wouldn't let us have a new toy triggered a spanking; and so on. After much repetition, trial and error, we began to recognize that inappropriate behaviors hurt other people, infringe on their rights, and in the long run threaten our own safety and well-being.

These early social tapes gradually change by association into images that are stored in our pictorial, holistic right hemisphere. As adults, these images have the power to trigger specific reactions.

For an example of how this works, take a look at Figure 1. Which of the two images best corresponds to your idea of "danger?"

Most of us would choose (A) as depicting the more "dangerous" situation. However, if we have stepped on or been cut by

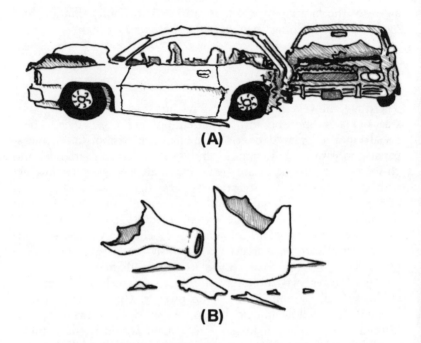

(A)

(B)

Figure 1 (A) & (B): Which of these two images
best corresponds to your idea of "danger"?

broken glass sometime in the past, we may connect (B) more
directly with danger — we have been "programmed" to do so.

Similarly, which of the pictures in Figure 2 corresponds to
your idea of "satisfaction?"

This time, the choice may be more difficult because both pictures evoke good feelings. But for some of us, the connection
between food and comfort was so strong during childhood that
we flash a mental image of food at the mere mention of the word
"satisfaction," even if no pictures are provided.

This indicates the kind of power that some of these subconscious images can have. Though their messages were appropriate
and helpful to us as children, as adults they often lead us to inappropriate responses in different situations. The examples we dis-

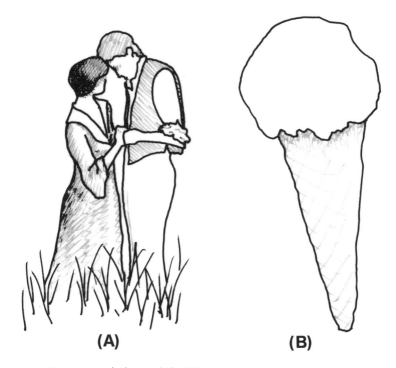

(A)　　　　　　　　**(B)**

Figure 2 (A) & (B): Which of these two images best corresponds to your idea of "satisfaction"?

cussed in Chapter 3 illustrate this clearly. Once the right brain stores images and feelings connected with an experience — a raised eyebrow; an angry tone of voice; the sweet taste and smooth texture of ice cream accompanied by laughter and sunny days at the beach — it recalls these images subconsciously in similar situations. That is how social tapes become mental tapes.

"Okay," you may be saying to yourself, "so what has all this to do with my being overweight? After all, I already know how I put on that fat — my mental tapes play messages like 'Eat this, you'll feel better' whenever I'm upset. Who cares whether some of my *mental* tapes were once *social* tapes?"

Nobody would care if these social tapes weren't still playing away. But the fact is, they are: New messages about food constantly bombard us from the media and even from our best friends, as they recycle *their* old childhood tapes and new social tapes. And these new tapes "out there" are eager to get "in here" and mess around with our right-brain images and our subconscious minds. All well and good when the new message is "Drive 55 and stay alive" (or face a costly speeding ticket). But what about tapes like "Show him you love him. Put Mother's Cookies in his lunch box tomorrow"?

Such messages greet us every day. Social tapes don't stop after we've reached age twenty-one, they are simply all those messages that keep competing for our attention as we pursue the very human activity of living with and trying to influence others. We need social tapes — they are an important means of communicating with one another. But let's listen to them and figure out what they're really saying to us. Let's be aware — and wary — of these never-ending messages from outside.

Because we are adults and have formed a certain number of reliable and trustworthy mental tapes of our own, we are more able to defend ourselves from inappropriate new social tapes than we were as children, when all we had to go on was parental tapes and our own visceral needs. Now that we've learned to cope with and interpret the world, we can bring our conscious awareness into play to evaluate the new messages we hear day in and day out.

There is, however, another factor that can cancel out our adult advantage: Society's messages seem to get more complicated, contradictory and confusing as time goes on. For example, let's take a look at some common social food tapes:

"Buy Fudgy-Wudgy Chocolate Cake Mix and show your family you love them." Sound familiar? This sort of social tape plays on the old theme of "love equals food," which we learned about in Chapter 3. Not many of us would *consciously* agree that we need to show our families we love them by baking them a chocolate cake, or even that the cake is necessarily good for them. Yet our old tapes that associate food with love may subconsciously agree with and accept the new message.

"When you don't have time to cook, grab a Fatburger at Burger Paradise." A couple of social tapes are in operation here. One of them reminds us that we live in a fast-paced, hurry-up culture in which time is not to be squandered on little-valued activities as cooking lean, nutritious meals. The other tape equates saving time (desirable) with eating "fast" — and often fat — food (which becomes desirable by association with the time savings). A double-whammy social tape if ever I heard one — and one to which I will devote more attention later in this chapter.

"Become thin and sexy and beautiful in only ten days with Chewy Caramel Appetite Suppressants." This sort of tape — which has had a pervasive influence on the values of our late-twentieth-century Western culture — really ups the ante. Now, all the things we'd really like to be or have — beauty, sexiness, and, by extension, love and happiness — are equated with being *thin*. But watch out, because here *thin* is equated with *food*. Indeed, this "beauty = thin = food" social tape is, I believe, the most dangerous and damaging of all. It encourages faulty thinking in two ways: first, by suggesting that our well-being depends on our being skinny, and second, by turning around and telling us that being skinny depends on eating something very like the kind of food that helped us to get fat in the first place. And this message is really mind-boggling when it starts to fight with the old "love = food" tape.

The notion that we can change our bodily form without changing our faulty eating behavior, that instead we should actually continue that behavior — substituting "diet" candy or a chocolatey, low-calorie liquid food supplement for the "real" thing — doesn't help one bit in maintaining and sustaining (let alone obtaining) our desired weight. In the second part of this book, I will have more to say about how we must change our attitudes and behavior toward food. First, let's examine that dominant social tape of twentieth-century Western culture: Thin equals beauty.

BEAUTY AND BODY WEIGHT

Throughout history and across cultures, body weight has been connected with beauty. Beauty, in turn, is connected with so many aspects of well-being — power, goodness, desirability, you name it — that it may well be the most sought-after component of happiness ever known. As a result, people pay a great deal of attention to social tapes concerning beauty.

Beauty is culturally determined. Over the course of history people have found beauty in fair or dark skin, in long or short hair, in scarification, jewelry, and other forms of bodily decoration — but never until now in emaciation.

"You can never be too rich or too thin" has become the received wisdom of the late twentieth century. We find women, especially, striving to be very, very thin. Thin enough for that size 6 dress, no matter what the woman's natural frame may dictate is best for her. We find little girls as young as five beginning to wonder in kindergarten whether those new designer jeans will make them look fat. Practically every woman with whom I have worked over the past ten years — even those who have never faced a significant weight challenge — is "struggling" with at least five pounds. Practically no woman today is pleased with her figure. How can she be when everything she sees and hears, especially from the media, sends out the social tape: Anything larger than a size 9 is definitely not in vogue, not even acceptable. What she needs to do, she keeps reading and hearing, is go on a diet, join a health club, become one of the "beautiful people." And the beautiful people are never fat. How many fat people do you see starring in today's daytime soaps, for example? Not too many.

So we have this mandate that we can never be too thin or too rich. How did this come about? When did this notion become an imperative, to the point where fourth- and fifth-grade girls are panicked if they gain two pounds? Why the bumpersticker NO FAT CHICKS? When did we become obsessed with being thin?

As we look through the history of how our ancestors viewed beauty in relationship to body weight, we find some interesting —

and startling — things. Venus de Milo was no "skinny chick." Botticelli's *The Birth of Venus* depicts a voluptuous nude whose belly and thighs, although well-proportioned in relation to the rest of her body, would be considered fat by today's standards. The great beauties painted by Michelangelo, da Vinci, Rembrandt, Renoir, Rubens, and a host of other artists are healthy, robust, and voluptuous. Madame Pompadour, the mistress of Louis XV, considered one of the most beautiful women of eighteenth-century France, would seem overweight to us. Yet such women as Madame Pompadour were considered desirable *because* of the fullness of their bodies.

We also find, in many different cultures, weight as a symbol of strength and prosperity. Henry VIII, for example, deliberately kept himself corpulent as a sign of his authority and power. Only those who could not afford to eat were thin; being skinny was definitely not "in." The images connecting thinness with poverty and disease, heftiness with wealth and health, were entrenched in our ancestors' right brains and remain so today in many parts of the world. In fact, this explains a lot of things: the ideal of beauty as voluptuousness, as well as the notion that the only healthy baby is a fat baby.

Although these standards are changing in Western cultures today, hefty or plump is still "in" in many parts of the world. Many Slavic men, for example, prefer their women full-bodied. I recently visited a friend from Hungary who was entertaining one of his countrymen. We enjoyed a wonderful evening together, with my friend acting as interpreter. As I was leaving, the Hungarian visitor made a comment to my friend, who laughed. I asked what he had said, but my friend tried to pass it off. When I persisted, he laughingly told me that his friend had commented that I was a pretty lady, but I had such "skinny crow legs" that it was a shame I couldn't fatten up a bit. He felt that I would look much more "smashing" with another twenty pounds on my body. Here I had jogged and worked out and faithfully watched my weight — only to be told that I was twenty pounds *under*weight! Beauty certainly is in the eyes of the beholder.

All cultures have different ideas of how beauty and body weight relate. In many cultures, the positive connection between heftiness and beauty results from the value those cultures place in healthy, strong women who can bear and rear the children so important to their livelihood. This Earth Mother ideal of feminine beauty stems from the importance of women as capable members of society, people who can "carry their own weight."

In the United States, similar ideals prevailed until the middle of this century. From the eighteenth century through the Great Depression, when most of our ancestors survived and prospered only through hard physical labor, health and beauty continued to be evidenced in full, well-proportioned bodies. Little thought was given to elaborate clothing styles or being thin simply to serve the whims of fashion. In the postindustrial period of the late nineteenth century, a few wealthy families — the Morgans, Vanderbilts, Rockefellers, and Astors — began to display their wealth by building huge, elaborate houses and by installing their women in those houses as "birds in gilded cages." For the first time in this society, a few women were mandated to abandon the Earth Mother, no-nonsense ideal and use their newfound leisure and labor-saving devices to become "child-women" who no longer needed to worry their pretty little heads about work. Paradoxically, though they were symbols of conspicuous consumption, these women were encouraged to stay small and thin. Cinched-in waists (remember Scarlett O'Hara?) were the rule. These women were as decorative — and as significant — as their husbands' watch fobs.

Nevertheless, they were still the exception. What about those women who were not among the chosen few, like our grandmothers and great-grandmothers? Most of them were still working the fields and the sweatshops. All they could do in the interests of fashion was to buy the magazines of their day, such as Godey's Lady's Book, and dream of how wonder-filled life must be in the Victorian mansions. The vast majority of women in America at the beginning of the twentieth century could live the gracious life only vicariously, through their limited knowledge of the upper class. Their own lives had no glamour at all; these hale and hearty working women had no-nonsense figures to go along with their no-nonsense lifestyles. Our grandmothers were interested in their wealthier counterparts, they enjoyed a sense of luxury in reading about their lives — and indeed, the tiny minority of wealthy, fashionable females touched off a yearning in the hearts of working women — but who had time for cinched-in waists?

And to speak truth, even these few wealthy nineteenth-century "star" women were not particularly thin. Lillian Russell, for example, was extremely popular, and she is said to have weighed 200 pounds. In the 1920s, Sophie Tucker and Mae West were voluptuous women, sporting "hour-glass" figures. During the 1930s we began to see women who were dainty and small-boned, yet still well-proportioned: Janet Gaynor, Bette Davis, and Gloria Swanson, for example. Next came the wartime, the 1940s, and paragons of beauty — Betty Grable, Esther Williams, Greer Garson, Greta Garbo, Carole Lombard — wore bathing suits that revealed nicely shaped, curved figures, with enough "meat" to provide the curves.

As recently as the 1950s — the so-called happy days — our movie sex goddesses carried full figures, and even today few men would deny the appeal of women like Jane Russell, Marilyn Monroe, or Jayne Mansfield. Many of us who were in high school and college during the 1950s wore crinoline petticoats (the more the better), poodle skirts down to our ankles (where our fluffy angora socks were rolled to perfection), and fluffy angora sweaters to match our socks. In short, we were not into looking thin. All those petticoats made even the slenderest among us look rather wide in the hips. Our bulky socks and saddle shoes and fluffy sweaters did nothing to help us look svelte.

IS BEAUTY "THIN" DEEP?

Given this history, one thing is clear: It was not until quite recently that our culture made the shift to "thin is in." And, for many of us, this new ethic of beauty has arisen within our lifetimes — as a new social tape, often in conflict with old mental tapes concerning beauty and self-worth.

Part of the trend toward emaciation may have started with clothing designers. In the 1950s and '60s, the fashion industry boomed in a sort of postwar marketing craze. Growing prosperity

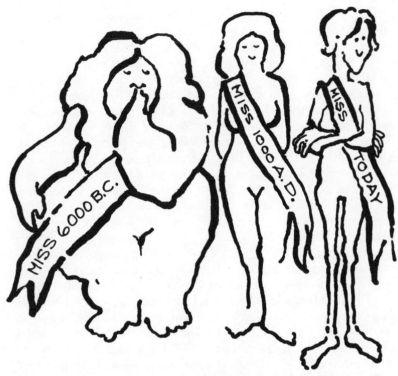

**It was not until quite recently that our culture made
the shift to "thin is in."**

invited growth in the production and purchase of consumer
goods — particularly clothing. Most designers of clothing for
women were men, as were the buyers who decided what mer-
chandise the department stores would stock and sell. *Haute cou-
ture* designers, preoccupied with the art of their creations, often
designed clothing that could be worn to advantage by only a tiny
minority of female figures — by women whose frames would not
detract from the "line" of the clothes. As these designs gained
status they were imitated and reproduced on a mass scale, for sale
to the majority of women. For the first time, women like you and
I could afford the clothes displayed in such high-fashion maga-

zines as Vogue and Harper's Bazaar. But our more voluptuous figures did not necessarily fit the clothes. Yet the models seemed to become ever-slimmer to fit the slimmer and slimmer attire. The 1960s focused on the glamour of Jackie O. and her lithe figure, on the women in those beach-party flicks who wore "itsy-bitsy, teenie-weenie, yellow polka-dot bikinis." In the rebellious 1960s — partly in protest against their parents' "establishment" way of life — young women aspired to the skinny body. Slimness became an ethic as well as a status symbol. Being skinny would enable women to wear all those spare garments — tight jeans, miniskirts, bikinis — that expressed a new sexual freedom. Paradoxically, the trend toward boyish figures also symbolized a new androgyny intended (at least indirectly) to deemphasize sexual differences and promote the cause of female freedom.

I am not knocking the values symbolized by these new bodily fashions — indeed, the social liberation that emanated from the 1960s is highly laudable. The problem is this: Fashion models, who wore the *symbols* of these new ethics to perfection, became *body* models for many, if not most, of us. To be "with it," we came to think that we had to look like them. Oh, maybe we didn't think so — consciously. But their figures, their images, became indelibly lodged in our pictorial right brains, and our subconscious minds proceeded to equate those images with beauty, sexiness, power, liberation — in short, with self-esteem.

By the time the 1970s and 1980s rolled around, we were a culture obsessed with our bodies. Expensive health spas sprouted up all over the country. We began to hear about a syndrome called *anorexia nervosa* (deliberate self-starvation) and then one call *bulimia* (deliberate food-bingeing accompanied by "purging," or self-induced vomiting). Pat Boone's daughter began to speak out publicly about anorexia nervosa, and we began to hear about more and more deaths, including that of singer Karen Carpenter, from this alarming condition. Even as early as the 1960s we had heard about the aftereffects of "diet" pills, which at one time were common in almost every woman's medicine cabinet and pill container. Judy Garland's tragic death forced many of us to reconsider the use of then-legal drugs for weight control. As the side effects of amphetamines began to be recognized, fad diets sprang up like toadstools, and we were exposed to a plethora of easily abused and often harmful means of "losing" weight: diet dust, liquid diets, crash diets, and so on. Take Off Pounds Sensibly (TOPS) was originally chartered in 1948, and Overeaters Anonymous and Weight Watchers followed in the 1960s. These three organizations recognized the dangers of these trends early on — while further characterizing our growing preoccupation with thinness.

What can we expect from the rest of the twentieth century? Not many of us today are drinking or popping diet pills. We are much more sophisticated now — much more "into" health — as evidenced by the emphasis on fitness and exercise. We are now tantalized not only by new diets but also by ads offering a full year's membership in a gym at half the "normal" price. So we "take advantage" of the offer and join an overcrowded spa that we end up never using. In other words, *we remain obsessed with our bodies and convinced that our well-being depends on our being thin.*

We are also in a big hurry. We live in a culture that demands instant gratification: instant foods, instant dry cleaning, instant enlightenment through training seminars that guarantee we'll get to the meaning of life in a few short sessions. I was in line at a fast-food place one day when the lady in front of me ordered some chicken and was told by the counterperson that the order would take a few minutes, since a new batch of chicken had just been put in the fryer. The customer asked just HOW LONG this might take. The server replied, "Between three and four minutes." The customer sighed, "Oh, all right, but hurry it up!" How in the world does one hurry up three minutes?

This ever-quickening pace brings with it, of course, the stress-related diseases and high divorce rates that are the by-products of our "life in the fast lane" age. It also helps to account for why we are overweight in a culture that seems to demand thinness. The average American meal is consumed in about seven minutes. I mean, from soup to nuts — burp! Consider the biological mechanism that tells us we're sated: The body, via the blood-sugar level, requires about twenty minutes to tell us we're full. No wonder so many of us eat more than we need. No wonder the restaurants serve portions at least twice the size necessary. We don't slow down enough to let our biochemistry tell us that we've had enough. We're too afraid that we might miss something good on television, or that we might have to sit there and interact with our families. We do not have the time for this nonsense; we have "bigger fish to fry."

What has happened is this: Our cultural image of the "idealized" self — the self our social tapes have told us is necessary for beauty, desirability, power, sexiness, happiness — and our "realized" selves — what we really are, including all of our individual physical idiosyncrasies — are worlds apart. On the one hand, the media tell us to eat at fast-food places, buy pizza, bake cookies for the family. On the other hand, there is a popular demand to be skinny in order to be "in" — to reject ourselves if we are anything less than "perfect," that is, anything other than what the current (faulty) social tapes demand.

Now, I am not advocating that we should try to become a fat nation. Even with all the social tapes that tell us we ought to be thin in order to be "actualized," we are still an overweight society. Approximately one out of every five Americans is clinically obese, and that is probably a conservative estimate. Yet to be fat today is not simply to be unhealthy but also (our social tapes tell us) a sign of weakness — a moral failing. The image of fat, which today goes beyond obviously unhealthy obesity to include anything more than five pounds over near-emaciation, has become associated in our right brains with ugliness, asexuality, moral lassitude, and sheer sinfulness. At the same time, eating remains associated with love and satisfaction, via our old childhood tapes. This fact is bound to produce a real schism in many people, particularly women.

FEAR OF SLIMNESS: GENDER TAPES

It always amazes me how women view their emotional involvement with fat. So many of them say that when they get thin — or even think of being thin — they get frightened. Why? When the culture dictates that being thin is in, why is this frightening?

Perhaps the answer lies in the assumption that once a woman is thin — and thus desirable and powerful — she has it "all together." And now that she has it all together, she is expected to perform. Many women I have interviewed and with whom I have worked therapeutically fear the great expectations that others might have of them. "If I get thin," these women say to themselves, "people will expect so much of me that I might not be able to perform. I might fall short of the standards they have set for me and imposed on me. Why bother with that diet? Forget it! Stay fat and safe — fat and unencumbered by the expectations of others."

There are subtle yet powerful fears that plague overweight women at the thought of being thin. Thin, in our culture, connotes sexy. Being thin therefore means that we are apt to exude sex, and males may take to the scent like hounds to fox. Now what? What to do with all this male attention? Where were all of these guys when I was twenty (or fifty or one hundred) pounds overweight? They weren't exactly breaking my door down then! Many of these women therefore feel some anger as well as fear — anger with both men and women — after reaching their desired weight. These formerly fat women feel that, while their men and women friends paid little or no attention to them when they were fat, now they "count" only because they have reduced their weight. Since they are still their "same selves," the change they perceive in others' behavior toward them is an understandable source of rage.

Many people who have attained their desired weight (perhaps by shedding a hundred pounds or more) experience this confusion. All of us depend, to a certain extent, upon the validation of others for our sense of self-identity. But we also have a strong self-image that continues despite dramatic changes in our physical appearance. Those of us who have rid ourselves of fat, believing that we are who we always were, cannot understand why our friends and acquaintances begin to respond differently to us. One woman told me that the fatter she got, the more invisible she became. When she reached her goal weight, however, she became visible. Now men stopped by her desk, chatted, made comments about how great she looked. She was so intimidated by all the attention and what it might demand of her that she regained the weight!

The emotions accompanying weight change present a real dilemma for the formerly fat person, and for some individuals that pressure may be devastating enough to cause them to put the weight back on. These people have not learned to understand and accept the reactions of others to their new bodies. When this happens, many formerly fat people fall back on old right-brain images that are laden with emotionality. They resort to the old patterns of solving their problems, and attempt to return to the status quo: fat.

I have also heard many women say that they regained their weight because they felt they were no longer taken "seriously" when they became thin. Somehow, they identified being thin with frivolous and vain behavior, which was inconsistent with their self-image. This self-image seems to be, to a large degree, a function of the right brain's pictorial activity. Whenever you and I perceive a conflict between our self-image in its idealized form and our self-image in its realized form, we begin to feel very uncomfortable. This conflict seems to happen for many women today.

How about the obese male? He, too, experiences conflict when he obtains his desired weight, but it often takes a different form. One of the most common complaints I have heard from men is that they seem to lose some of their authority; they do not feel that they can back up their demands or requests when their weight diminishes. Something in their belief system connects power with bigness, and many feel that they are not taken as seriously when they lose that bigness. Thus the saying, "He really throws his weight around." These men fear that being thin may indicate being weak and thus may interfere with their "macho" image.

Fewer males than females express a fear of being more sexual when they are thin. Still, I have heard some men, particularly younger men, express a related fear. One young man, who was very tall and handsome, told me that he was fearful of being rejected when asking a woman for a date. He had been very obese as a young child and had reduced his weight after his freshman year in high school. By his junior year, he was slim, and the girls were flirting with him. He gradually became less fearful and began to approach girls for dates.

All went well until he entered college and had his first sexual encounter. This man had a small penis for the size of his body. He had been concerned about this for some time, yet it had not posed a big problem until he became sexually active. During his first sexual encounter, his fear of how he would perform led to a failure to penetrate, and he vowed to date no more. Within six weeks after this encounter, he began to gain weight and quickly returned to his highest weight, which he had carried in the seventh grade. Gradually, he passed this level too, and when he came into therapy, he weighed more than 250 pounds. It took many months in therapy for him to consider that he could have a satisfactory friendship with a woman whom he really loved before he attempted sex. For this young man, so-called casual sex was hardly advisable; first he had to build up a trusting relationship with a woman. He has yet to find that "special someone," but at least he is looking and need not hide behind his fat for fear that he will not perform well sexually.

Some married men have another fear: that if they become too slim and trim, they will be tempted to go outside their marriage for sex. One gentleman with whom I worked was a salesman who traveled a great deal. After reducing his weight because of a medical problem, he suddenly found himself looking at other women and desiring to have relationships with them. We discussed this in therapy, and gradually he was able to sort out his feelings and consider how he wanted to handle these impulses. It isn't the impulse that counts; it is how we act on that impulse that breaks up marriages. He was able to discuss with his wife how he felt about having women look at him differently now that he was thin for the first time in thirteen years. She was able to work with him on the issue, and they are still happily married today.

OVERCOMING FEAR:
REFORMING RIGHT-BRAIN SELF-IMAGES

We see, then, that both men and women experience conflicting emotions and uneasiness when they approach their desired weight. Sometimes these conflicts are so threatening that the overweight person will look in the mirror and not even notice his fat. Studies have shown that overweight people tend to use a mirror only under necessary conditions — to comb their hair, shave, brush their teeth, and so on. When these people do look in the mirror, they tend to look only at their faces. They rarely look below their necks and almost never scan their bodies. A type of self-denial is in operation here, a sort of "What I don't see can't exist."

On the other hand, there are those people who begin to approach their desired weight and fail to see their bodies changing. Even though the scales and the mirror accurately reflect changes in their bodies, their right-brain, visual side does not accept what their eyes see. Many people who are approaching their desired weight tell me that, although all of their friends have commented that their bodies are looking great, they truly do not see change occurring. They lament that although others see them as thin, they themselves still see a fat person when they look in the mirror. This distorted body image is quite common among fat people who are shedding weight. Perhaps it stems from being large for a long time and being used to looking that way. That is, the right brain may persist in visualizing the body as overweight. This common problem poses a two-edged danger: The individual may continue to lose weight in order to reach an ever-diminishing goal (the syndrome known as anorexia nervosa) or, on the contrary, the individual may become disillusioned by the "failure" of his attempts, give up altogether and return to comforting patterns of overeating.

An old therapeutic "trick" for dealing with this adjustment problem is to cut out a picture of a person with a thin body and paste a photo of the fat person's face over it. This technique tends to "fool" the right brain, which begins to agree with the image it sees. The individual's holistic, right-brain, subconscious side accepts the new image and begins to focus on it. Because the subconscious mind is a servile mechanism, accepting what the conscious mind tells it, it acts as if the picture were true — or at least believable.

FIT NOT THIN

What are we to do? How do we begin to reconcile the conflicting ideals in our belief systems? It seems that the trends toward obesity, anorexia nervosa, and bulimia will continue until we can begin to shift toward realistic body images. How do we do that? Each of us must learn to take personal responsibility for his or her own health. This includes moving down the healthy road to obtaining, maintaining, and sustaining our desired weight. And "desired" does not have to mean "skinny." We must be centered enough to recognize the difference between what we see "out there" in the media and what is right for us, and accept our bodies at their normal weights. To strive for rail-thinness is as ridiculous as it is to strive to be a hundred pounds overweight.

Our body weight reflects our thinking process, which in turn is influenced by what our culture's social tapes tell us. But we are adults, after all: We can decide for ourselves what weight is appropriate — and healthy — for us. Making that decision is what the next chapter is all about.

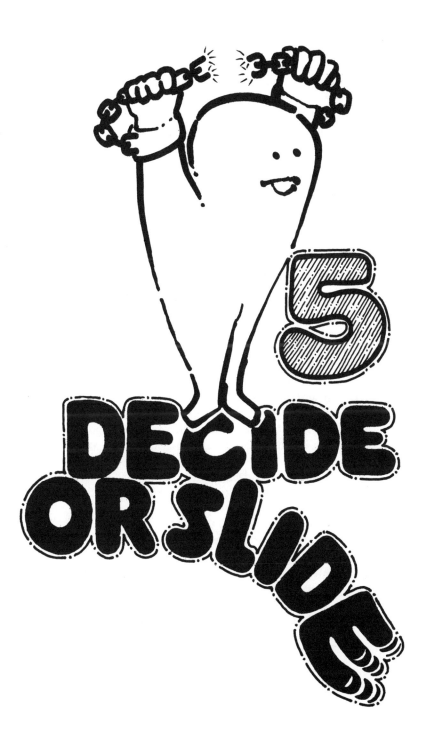

5

DECIDE OR SLIDE

Dear Fat,

You have shielded me from the outside world...
made me look big and strong and able to take care of
myself. You have protected me from people who wanted
"only my body" and have forced me to meet them only
on an intellectual level. You have sheltered me and
comforted me when everyone hated me. Well, they
hate me because of you. Because of you, they think I
am ugly and lazy and worthless. Maybe I am. But you
were always there to take my mind off tears and
sadness. I'll never be one of the beautiful people... I
can't write anymore...

IN CHAPTER ONE, I SET OUT THE BASIC TENET OF THIS BOOK:
Fat is in consciousness. Fat is, for many of us, directly linked to
our subconscious learned behaviors. We find ourselves fat because
somewhere we learned faulty problem solving. When we reach for
a Tootsie Roll in order to feel better, that's faulty problem
solving.

When you and I learn to bring some of these faulty problem-
solving behaviors to conscious awareness, then we can begin to
learn new ways to solve problems. In fact, our "problems" become upgraded to challenges — challenges that we can tackle in
ways that are healthy and that lead to our desired weight. Ulti-
mately, it is up to us to *decide* either to focus on new ways of
meeting emotional challenges or to *slide* back into our old habits
of eating to reduce tension.

You and I must take a stand: DECIDE OR SLIDE. Which
will it be? If we choose to decide, our need is to learn new
behaviors. In the following chapters, you will learn how to incorporate new behaviors into your life. For now, start by making the
decision to concentrate on changing those old childhood tapes
from Chapter 3, and the current social messages about food
which we have just discussed in Chapter 4. Your conscious decision to do so is the key to replacing them with mature, adult
alternatives for handling stress in constructive ways.

THE NEW PARADIGM: SELF-RESPONSIBILITY

If we review some of the trends in our culture, we find that this idea of making a conscious decision to change our attitudes is coming into vogue. John Naisbitt, for example, in his best-seller *Megatrends*, observes that people are becoming increasingly involved with their health, and this naturally includes attitudes toward weight. More and more, people are realizing that playing a passive role in the control of their body weight just doesn't work.

Traditionally, we have turned to health professionals (physicians, psychologists, and so on) to help us face health challenges. We have run to our doctors and asked them to give us something or do something to us in order to get us to our "ideal" weight. We have taken shots, consumed pills, and even taken extreme measures such as surgery to "lose" weight. All of these activities are passive: We wait to see what "they" are going to do about our weight. Today, this attitude is changing, as are many other ideas about self-care.

Marilyn Ferguson, in her book *The Aquarian Conspiracy*, also addresses what she calls the "new paradigm" in health care. A paradigm is a way of explaining reality. Patients are no longer passive recipients of health care, they are becoming more directly involved, not only with decisions regarding their health but also with actual procedures. The patient-doctor relationship is beginning to realign. Now it's more of a fifty-fifty proposition.

Naturally, the skilled professional retains a great responsibility for correctly identifying the various causes of health problems and recommending possible courses to follow for treatment or remediation. Yet, more and more, the physician looks to the patient to follow through on his or her own. One example: For many years physicians have cautioned people to stop smoking, reduce their weight, work at less stressful jobs, and take other steps to ensure better health. Today it has become clear that unless the patient is a partner in this endeavor, nothing happens. I believe that "tuitioned" people (those who are begged, cajoled, threatened, or manipulated into changing) do very poorly. They eventually go back to their original faulty ways of meeting their health challenges. The initiative must come from us, the patients.

So it is with the obese person. Overweight people must be willing to take personal responsibility for their weight. They must be willing to answer the physician's question regarding what *they* intend to do about their weight. The physician or psychologist is a partner in the process, but the ultimate responsibility lies with each individual.

This may seem harsh or callous at first, but stop to think about it for a minute. You see, if we rely on others to do things for us, we render ourselves helpless. We become passive subjects rather than active partners in pursuit of a goal that is in our own best interest. When patient and physician view the goal of achieving a desired weight as the *patient's* responsibility, with the doctor as head coach and cheerleader, the chances of a positive outcome are greatly improved. When weight reduction is the *physician's* idea and responsibility, even though the patient's health may be in danger, the individual tends to regain weight because he or she has no stake in the action.

The same is true of the psychotherapist and the obese patient. Many people have come to me and lamented that they want to reduce their weight but just cannot seem to do it. One of the first questions I ask them is, "Are you committed to achieving and keeping your desired weight?" People must know at the outset that they are the principals in the procedure. The therapist may guide, suggest, and support, but it is the individual who must play the lead role in the process.

Truly, we must decide or slide. We either decide to change and follow the guidelines set by the physician or psychotherapist, or we slide back into old patterns of passive resistance. To be successful, the process must be a *conscious* one.

This trend toward self-responsibility had its beginnings in the 1970s, when many of today's so-called self-help groups — est, Actualizations, Life Spring, and countless others — were established. The trend is reflected in every aspect of our culture. Industry and management picked up on the idea and developed it into "quality circles" and "Theory Y" management. The teaching and sales professions also saw the value of stressing self-responsibility. Multilevel marketing corporations sprung up like mushrooms, touting the importance of self-responsibility and accountability, of being a "self-starter." You may have as much wealth and success as you are willing to work for.

And so we find that this basic psychological principle is alive and well in the modern psychotherapist's attitude toward weight. The individual, herself or himself, must be deeply involved in the process. No blaming or shaming of yourself or others. No more "I'm fat because of my genes" or "I'm fat because of a hormonal deficiency" or "I'm fat because my parents overfed me" or even "I'm fat because he makes me so mad I have to eat." These are no longer culturally acceptable paradigms. Today, psychotherapists prefer to head off our need to blame or shame others by helping us learn better methods of assessing where the responsibility for our weight really lies. The concept of self-responsibility is essential if we are truly to obtain, maintain, and sustain our desired weight for as long as we choose to do so.

In keeping with this mandate of accountability comes a change in the reasons people give for allowing themselves to be fat. If, as the statistics almost always tell us, fat is rarely caused by a genetic predisposition alone, then what *is* the cause of fat? Once we rule out hormonal imbalances and external influences as common reasons for obesity, then what reason is left?

This is where the concept of self-responsibility applies so well. When other avenues are closed, we come face-to-face with ourselves. And as we confront ourselves, we become aware that, just maybe, *we* have some connection with our own fat. After all, we must have done something to get it; it wasn't *given* to us. Unlike a dramatic heart attack, people rarely have a "fat attack" as they are walking down the street! It just doesn't work that way!

This is not to say, of course, that certain people do not have a greater predisposition to being fat than others. There are people who have inherited a tendency toward obesity, and members of the same family also have a tendency to carry their fat in the same places. Yet a *tendency* toward fat rarely causes a person to *remain* fat. Such people may find their weight a greater challenge than most, but very few are genetically doomed to be fat. I have worked with many individuals who came from fat families and felt they were doomed. But then they learned new thought patterns and now know that this is not so. Many of these people have remained at their desired weight for years after they learned to change their subconscious behavior and conscious thinking with regard to food.

EMOTIONS: THE EFFECT OF AFFECT

Along with the emphasis on self-responsibility, there is a shift from an intellectual to an affectual (or emotional) approach in weight management. More and more, psychotherapists and physicians are realizing that obesity has an emotional base that does not respond to intellectual processes.

Not long ago, a big-city newspaper reported a study in which researchers showed a group of kindergarten children a picture of a fat child and a "normal" child (the researchers' word, not mine) and asked what the differences were between the two children. Ninety-three percent of these five-year-olds said that the main difference between the children was that one was fat and the other was not. When asked why the one child was fat, more than 90% responded that the child ate too much. As we may conclude from these youngsters' observations, the origin of fat is no intellectual mystery. Most five-year-old children can come up with the commonsense reason for obesity: People are overweight because they overeat. Why, then, has our culture persevered in treating obesity as if it were an intellectual, rational problem?

The rational approach is, of course, the basis of dieting. Just get on a good diet and stick to it. Sound logic. Just stay on a diet until you get to your "ideal" weight and you'll be fine. Solid concept. Just eat less and exercise more and you'll lose weight. Again, great cognitive approach. As we all know from experience, however, these intellectual, cognitive approaches just don't work. If they did, we would all push ourselves away from the table as the physicians keep telling us to, and we would all be thin. But we aren't. Every time you lose weight through deprivation, your cycle turns to the reward phase and your "lost" weight quickly reappears. Fat cells never go away. They merely shrink up and lie

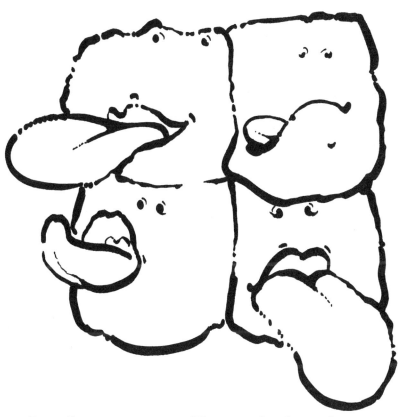

Fat cells never go away. They just lie there, dormant, waiting for you to reward yourself...

there, dormant, just waiting for you to reward yourself so they can spring back into action!

There are countless volumes on weight control and dieting — all offering guaranteed, surefire, keep-it-off-forever routines. And most of these books use an intellectual, left-brain, reasonable approach. Perhaps they are missing the point. Maybe the medical and psychological communities are failing to recognize one essential component of the weight problem: feelings. We must bring into consciousness the old emotions and past programming that keep prompting today's overeating.

The subconscious mind is very tricky, subtle, and powerful, but it can be harnessed. As you learned in Chapters 3 and 4, we need to bring to conscious light some of the information stored in the subconscious. Once we do this, we can begin to obtain, maintain, and sustain our desired weight — for life! No longer do we need to blame our genes, our parents, or our spouses for our fat. Today's paradigm shift toward accountability challenges us to meet our fat personally.

Naturally, we will still have the support of our health professionals in our endeavors, but it is up to us to make the proper decision to reach our desired weight. There's a saying: "If it's to be, it's up to me." Nowhere is this more true than in the context of weight management.

NOTICE — DON'T JUDGE

A word of caution here: Sometimes we translate self-responsibility into self-blame. No. Definitely NO! Blame misses the point entirely. Self-responsibility implies that we have the power to change. Self-blame implies failure. Self-responsibility does not mean attacking ourselves when we gain insight into our personalities; otherwise the source of that insight will dry up. Self-responsibility means simply noticing our part in our weight and accepting it, recognizing that there are many productive avenues we can take to change it.

That is why I use the word "notice": We notice our responsibility for our weight. Notice is a far cry from "evaluate." We already evaluate our behavior constantly, and we generally end up criticizing ourselves. So the main issue here is to notice, to observe the behavior that leads us toward obesity. In noticing, we do not judge. Chronic blaming and shaming of ourselves only leads to further weight gain.

We've all been on guilt trips. The more we blame ourselves, the more guilty we feel and the more tension we experience. And as we experience greater tension, we gravitate back toward the old way of reducing tension: eating. We play all those old tapes again.

What we must learn is to detach ourselves from evaluating our behavior. Later chapters will give you the "how to" exercises that will help you learn this process. For now, please do just one thing: observe your behavior, but do not evaluate it as good or bad, evil or noble. Simply practice *noticing your behavior.*

Those of us who blame and shame ourselves for being "fat slobs" feel that we have sinned against ourselves or let all those people down who are cheering us on. "Sin" is an interesting word. It is connected with an old archery term meaning "to miss the mark." This is good news for those of us who have "sinned" by overeating: perhaps all we have done is to miss the mark. Once we learn new patterns of awareness, we sin no more, and we make our mark for ourselves!

As we move away from old feelings of guilt and blame about our weight, and toward new feelings of self-responsibility and mastery, we usually begin to feel free of that old obsessive need to eat. It is paradoxical, but the more we give ourselves permission to make occasional mistakes without severe reprimands, the more confident we become about being able to handle food nonabusively.

PAIN-CHAIN EATING

The old feelings of guilt and self-blame lead to what I call the "pain chain" of eating behavior. The pain-chain theory came out of one of my weight management groups, when it became clear to me that there is a predictable circular pattern to weight gain, and that this vicious cycle is definitely tied to emotional aspects of the obese individual's personality.

The pain-chain cycle goes something like this: I have an emotion (usually a subconscious one). I feel uneasy. I begin to search for relief. I turn to something that I have learned in the past will be a surefire cure for the tension: I get some food. Now, curiously enough, I feel momentary relief. I say "momentary," because very soon relief is followed by a stronger, more demeaning feeling: guilt. Then I start asking myself, "Why did I do that?" I admonish myself. I wasn't really hungry, and now I feel worse than ever. I'm ashamed and remorseful, and I'm afraid that someone will notice the missing ice cream. Quick, off to the store for a replacement! Musn't let anyone know I failed again. Then, after all the guilt and self-blame, I turn to another astonishing behavior — anger at myself, which may quickly turn to self-disgust, which starts the pain chain over again. "What the heck, I already blew my diet, so I might as well polish off the whole carton of ice cream. I have to replace it anyhow, so why not?"

We usually slide into this kind of reasoning after raging against ourselves. We're giving in, but we're also angry. It's the rebellious child within us yelling, "I'll show you!" First we punished ourselves with self-recrimination. Now we punish ourselves some more. This is truly a vicious cycle, and most of us find it too close to the truth for comfort.

Well, maybe one chocolate cookie will put a dent in our weight management program, but a whole package will blow it to kingdom come! So we need to examine our illogical thought process: "What the heck, I blew my diet already, so I might as well finish off the entire package." We can't stem the tide of this faulty logic until we really begin to notice the emotions and thoughts that led to the self-destructive behavior in the first place. Only then can we begin to deal with them directly and constructively.

Exercise

Right now, I'd like you to try a simple exercise. Don't worry, I'm not talking aerobics (yet). Finish this sentence:

"Being fat is _____."

Do it as quickly as you can, approximately ten times. Don't stop to think it through intellectually; just let yourself free-associate.

_____

_____

_____

_____

_____

Now see if any of the following statements — which come from former members of my weight management groups — rings a bell for you:

Being fat is wearing a coat when it isn't cold.

Being fat is sitting at the back of the auditorium, even if you can't hear.

Being fat is always having to shop at Omar the Tent-Maker's.

Being fat is sitting in the audience praying that your ticket number will not be called for the prize.

Being fat is never being able to eat an ice cream cone in public.

Being fat is never saying no.

Being fat is being jolly — no matter what.

Being fat is being asexual.

Being fat is always sitting in the aisle seat (so you don't have to squeeze in front of people).

Being fat is telling the checkstand person that the cake is for a friend's birthday.

BREAKING FREE: A CASE STUDY

You can see that "being fat" means different things to different people. The anonymous "Dear Fat" letter at the beginning of this chapter tells how one young woman felt about her fat. To protect her privacy, I'll call her Jean. Her story serves as an excellent example of how each of us must decide or slide, and how self-responsibility is the key to obtaining, maintaining, and sustaining our desired weight for life.

I chose Jean as an example because I have seen her in many group sessions as well as in individual sessions for psychotherapy. Her life story is of interest to any compassionate person. She had a childhood which rivals that of the multiple personality portrayed in Flora Rheta Schreiber's book *Sybil.*

Jean was an only child. Her mother was morbidly obese (more than twice her normal body weight) for most of her life. Her father was a mild-mannered man who was chained to the whims of his strong, large, manipulative wife. Jean remembers vividly being very, very little (probably before year one) and being in her crib when someone brought her a warm bottle of milk. She has great memories of how good it tasted and how secure she felt with her blanket as she drank it. Her years as a toddler, however, are generally a blank, and her first graphic memory of being alive after the stage of infancy is when she was in kindergarten. She recalls having to rush home after morning kindergarten to care for her mother, who was bedridden due to her extreme obesity (and probably because of psychotic episodes). From kindergarten until she left home at age fifteen, Jean's life was truly a living nightmare.

Jean's mother began accusing her of doing "nasty things" with men at a very young age. Such an idea is, of course, completely foreign to a young mind. Jean was soon taught, however, that "men are all alike — they're after only one thing." Repeated beatings (many of them so brutal that she couldn't go to school for days) and accusations of being a whore and a slut played throughout her childhood. Jean recalls her father's feeble attempts to intervene, but his protests only made the next day's beating worse. Finally, Jean and her father got the picture: There was no hope. He was too weak and involved in protecting himself to protect his young daughter, and Jean was too young to defend herself. They both gave in to the tyrant.

Finally, just after her fifteenth birthday, Jean received a beating that left her deaf in one ear and partially paralyzed in one arm for months. She ran from home with only the clothes on her back. A neighbor got her to a church, and the church placed her in a safe home for a year. After that, she was on her own. And now, for the first time, she began to get fat. It amazed her, but it didn't stop her overeating. Soon she met an older man who abused her and left her pregnant. She had the child alone in a charity hospital in Los Angeles.

When Jean and I first met, she was thirty and had managed to establish herself as a professional secretary, thanks to her intelligence and, surprisingly, her good nature. At this point she weighed about 350 pounds and was feeling strong and able to take care of herself. The following "Dear Fat" letter shows how she learned to feel about herself after she had been in therapy for eight months — much more positive, compared with her letter at the beginning of this chapter:

Dear Fat,

You were my insulation from the world. Fat people aren't expected to do a lot of things or succeed. Men don't come on to fat women, so I didn't have to deal with that. You were my excuse for not participating in my own life. That is no longer true. I'm removing this wall of fat I have built over the years. A wall works two ways: It may keep out things that hurt, but it also keeps out many things that I want. You have been my only "one" — you never left me alone like others in my life. But because you were there, there was no one else. Now you are being replaced by thin and people.

At first, I doubted I could do the Reflective Relearning process and affirm over and over to myself that I could obtain, maintain, and sustain my desired weight. I just did like she [the therapist] said, and after about two weeks I could tell the difference. I guess it's true what she keeps saying about "fake it till you make it." I lacked the confidence that I could really let go of fat, which had seemed to make me feel secure. But now, as I have replaced those tapes in my head, I feel really very confident that I finally have control over my bingeing and head-hunger eating. This feeling of control is the greatest thing I have ever experienced in my life. I intend to continue my ten minutes of self-talk daily. So far, it has been eight months and 105 pounds and about thirty-five hours total of Reflective Relearning time. I feel like my subconscious mind and my right brain are on MY side for the first time in my life. I am 131 pounds and love me. I'm worth the ten minutes a day!

Jean and I spent many, many hours finding out how her childhood beatings had compelled her to feel that she needed to be big and strong so she could defend herself from abusive men. Jean could now begin to make some decisions about her life. For example, she was heavily involved in an affair with her superior at work, and he was making unreasonable sexual demands upon her. She was appalled by them. Gaining therapeutic insight, she was learning to put together parts of the puzzle and make some different decisions.

Jean has now decided that she can and will find sanctuary in her own personal strength. She has decided to take charge of her own life. She has begun to see that blaming her mother is futile, since her mother was obviously psychotic. Blaming her neurotic father has also proved to be a dead end. There is another saying I'd like to share with you: "For what my parents did to me in the past, they are responsible; for what I do to myself from this day forward, I am responsible." Jean is now taking personal responsibility for what she does to herself. It has been a long, slow road, and she is still working on her relationship with her teenage son (who is also quite obese). But she is now within five pounds of her desired weight — a change of more than 100 pounds — and is happier than ever before in her life. She is learning to define and trust her own sense of self.

Jean's determination to stop sliding and start deciding was the key to her new life. Once she fully experienced the joy of taking personal responsibility for her life, no matter how unfortunate her past, she was in control. Sure, she still struggles with wanting to reach for a candy bar to "feel better." But she has a new inner strength. She practices her Reflective Relearning exercises daily, and she still occasionally calls me for some guidance. For the most part, she has directed her life and is dedicated to deciding and not sliding.

Chances are that you have never had the tremendous emotional challenges that Jean has faced in her life. Compared to her experiences, yours and mine may seem insignificant. Jean is truly a great model for anyone faced with the process of taking responsibility and making a commitment to self.

Remember, we can all occasionally fall prey to pain-chain eating behavior. When that happens, don't give up. Instead, *forgive yourself* and build a better plan for next time. "Next time" is the key, not "Now look what you have done, you fat pig." Jean and others who have suffered traumatic events set sterling examples for all of us. We must discover within ourselves what "being fat" is, and address the answer with determination.

The future promises to be an age of more and more personal accountability for our lives, as well as more responsibility for the lives of others on the planet. Self-responsibility in this context means the ability to see far enough ahead to set new plans. And that's what you are about to do in the next two chapters.

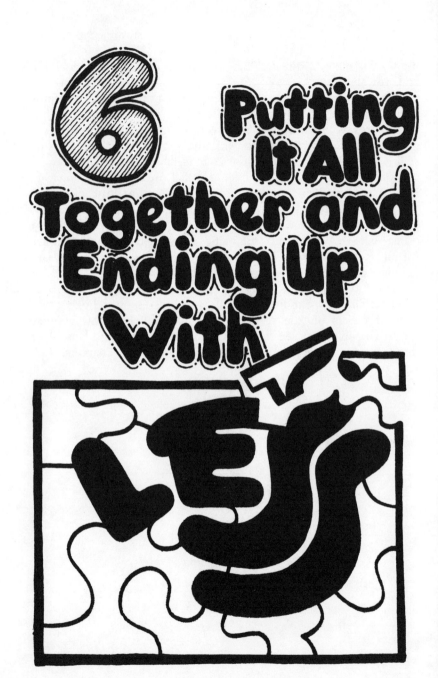

6 Putting It All Together and Ending Up With

NOW IT'S TIME FOR US TO PUT IT ALL TOGETHER and end up with less (fat, that is). We have learned how early childhood conditioning can lead to overeating, driving us to "eat this and feel better." We have also seen how social tapes have contributed to the complex phenomenon we call "obesity." For most of us, these social messages insist that we can never be too rich or too thin, while at the same time television commercials urge us to stop by the local fast-food place, where the food is not as F-A-S-T as it is simply F-A-T.

For most overweight people, fat is the result of the faulty problem solving that stems from these now-subconscious messages. We learned to reach for food when we are frustrated or emotionally challenged in some way. Somewhere deep in our right brain, the images that connect "filling full" with "fulfillment" continue to prompt the automatic, subconscious tape, "Eat this and make all the hurt go away." Our logical left brain would tell us that this message is ridiculous, but because we haven't allowed the left brain to become consciously aware of what the right brain is doing, we continue to reach for food as the way of "solving" our problems.

The old, traditional ways of "losing" weight are no longer appropriate, either. Dieting doesn't work, and we all know it! Diets are based on deprivation-reward systems that produce circular, rather than progressive, behavior patterns. No wonder we become discouraged and throw up our hands in despair, yelling that we were born to be fat! We are driven to believe our own rationalizations and self-deceptions, perhaps even obviously absurd ones, such as "If God didn't want me to be fat, He wouldn't have invented chocolate!"

We also know that pills, shots, surgery, and other medical interventions are no longer the treatment of choice. The idea that doctors are responsible for our health is no longer accepted in today's culture (and, in fact, never was very practical). Instead, self-responsibility is the byword, and back-to-basics the motto of our time. We no longer rely solely on the medical community to solve our problems in the Santa Claus tradition. We are no longer passive recipients of our health care — including our weight management. We recognize that our active cooperation, our participation and involvement in our own well-being is vital. After all, physicians can prescribe a nutritional plan, but they are not responsible if we do not follow it.

THE ANSWERS WITHIN

Related to this "back-to-basics" idea is our new-age tendency to turn inward for guidance rather than reach out like helpless children lost in the forest. On one level, fat is no big intellectual mystery. We all know how we got fat. But maybe we're still confused about *why* we did it, and the answer to that question usually comes as much from the inside as from the outside. So one of the basics we need to get back to is our inner wisdom.

The ancients knew this wisdom as something related to "divine inspiration" — the ability to grasp the core or truth of things. Poets have called it the Muse, and creativity is closely associated with this inner wisdom. How often have you scratched your head over a baffling problem, finally resolving to set it aside for a while or "sleep on it"? Comes the morning, and suddenly comes the dawn, too. You wake up to a solution that is now amazingly clear, as though someone out there had served it up on a silver platter (excuse the food imagery). "Why didn't I see it before?" you sometimes wonder.

Today, as we learn more about the right brain and the subconscious mind, we are discovering that this process is less mysterious than it appears. The answers aren't "out there," they are *within* us. We now know that the right brain and the subconscious mind play a constant, vital role in our thought patterns and daily behavior. As we have seen, their power can result in faulty problem solving. But that same power can be channeled into appropriate, constructive thoughts and actions. In order to tap this inner wisdom and make it work for us, we must learn to allow ourselves the privilege of being alone with ourselves. We need to look for answers within. This looking and listening within will strengthen our lives in countless ways. Not only will our desired weight start to manifest itself, but other health-enhancing life patterns will emerge — if we are diligent.

We can start by making a conscious, intellectual decision to *do* something. Remember the decision we made after reading Chapter 5, "Decide or Slide"? That was the all-important first step. The DO-DO principle works every time. Stop wishful thinking and start doing: *Do* give yourself the grand total of ten minutes per day to teach yourself how you expect to be. Not what you *want* to be, but how you *expect* to be. We do not always get what we want in life, but we nearly always get what we expect in life.

The self-caring person sees the value of using preventive measures to ensure desired weight. Therefore, daily ten-minute sessions become a must, not only to allow you to get to your goal, but also to keep you at your goal by preventing negative, faulty thinking from clouding your judgment. Using this preventive approach to weight control means that you take all your wishing and trying and self-blaming and upgrade them to direct intentions and expectations.

Diligent efforts pay off. Good intentions may pave the way to you-know-where, but that's only when they lack the determination of expectation. Intention without expectation doesn't get us very far. Once we expect a change in our lives, however, the change, as far as our thinking goes, is already an accomplished fact. All that's left to make the expectation a reality is time and adherence to a plan.

THE WRITE WAY: KEEPING A JOURNAL

Alright, now for the "how to." Beginning in this chapter, and continuing to more advanced levels in the next two chapters, I offer a plan for getting in touch with your right brain and subconscious mind.

Here, I'm going to start you out slowly. In the remainder of this chapter, we will concentrate on a very simple technique for getting in touch with our feelings on a daily basis: keeping a journal. This exercise is one that most newcomers to the Reflective Relearning technique will find comfortable and nonthreatening, for it allows us to approach our right-brain and subconscious thinking through the familiar "front door" of the conscious, verbal left brain. For those of us who have been "away from" or completely unaware of our right-brain, emotional side, a notebook offers something tangible and concrete for us to grasp — a sort of rational buoy as we start to tread subconscious waters. Keeping a journal allows our left brain to "do" something it can understand while we approach our right-brain, subconscious thoughts. In Chapter 7, you will really begin to "swim" as you dive into the Reflective Relearning experience. Keeping a journal now will prepare you for that experience and, what's more, will provide a repository for your left-brain, logical responses to the right-brain, subconscious experiences you will go through later on.

For now, then, your left brain is "getting off easy" as we allow it to participate in our initial contact with the right. Remember, *weight is in consciousness*, which means *awareness*. The more aware and conscious we become, the more control we have over the obsessive behavior of overeating.

To keep a journal, the first thing you need to do is get a notebook. Get one with at least enough pages to last six weeks, preferably with lined paper. Find one in which you'll enjoy writing. Perhaps a pleasant cover will be inviting. You may even enjoy investing some time designing your own cover; if so, try creating a design that reflects the purpose of your notebook — or any pattern of colors and shapes that appeals to you. Likewise, you may wish to select a few inexpensive felt-tip pens of various colors to write with, switching colors as your moods dictate. After all, this experience is for you. You are working to make your life more enjoyable, and the creativity you bring to the process can be as much fun as reaching the goal itself.

Keep your notebook by your bed, or close to wherever you can find a quiet spot where you can write, undisturbed, for ten minutes every day. If you're afraid that others may read your notebook, hide it in a safe place. Hide it between the mattress and the box springs — unless someone turns your mattress daily! Hide it wherever you feel secure that it will not be discovered. Many people feel uneasy that others may learn their innermost thoughts, and use that as an excuse for not committing their feelings to paper. Well, it's a feeble excuse. Anyone can find at least one hiding place that's safe from invasion.

THE OBJECTIVE REPORTER:
GETTING TO KNOW YOURSELF

A more realistic fear, common to many of us, is that of having to face our own thoughts and emotions in writing. This fear is similar to the tendency of overweight people (discussed in Chapter 4) to avoid surveying their bodies in a full-length mirror — a sort of self-denial. The feelings we record in a journal can act as a verbal mirror, reflecting back to us not only our attitudes about life in general and our feelings toward others but also our opinions of ourselves. Since many overweight people experience negative self-attitudes, they prefer not to have to confront those feelings, at least not directly.

Let me emphasize here that the very point of keeping a journal is to learn about our emotions, especially our feelings about ourselves. It is not, however, intended to be an exercise in self-denial or self-hate. We cannot "hate away" our fat. In fact, the more we hate our fat (and hence ourselves, since fat is currently a part of us), the longer it seems to hang around. You must accept yourself as you are today, in a body that is currently part of you. You are, after all, much more than your excess poundage — you are a person who values himself or herself enough to read this book and make an effort to enhance your life. Deep down, then, you must have a fairly good opinion of yourself, and indeed you should.

For this reason, I will impose only one rule upon your journal-writing: *Observe, but do not judge.* This means that you aren't allowed to use words such as "good," "bad," "stupid," "hate," and so on. Report your eating behavior for the day passively — do not put passion into it. Please do not write, "I pigged out and now I hate myself."

This is a difficult rule to follow — don't kid yourself! The left brain is not only our verbal side, it is our critical, evaluative, judgmental side, and it will insist, over and over, that you should analyze, draw conclusions from, and form an opinion of your behavior. But there are opinions, and then there are opinions. When you've polished off the last of that half-gallon of ice cream after a tough day at work your left brain can choose to form several opinions. One might be: "You are a weak, gutless, fat slob,

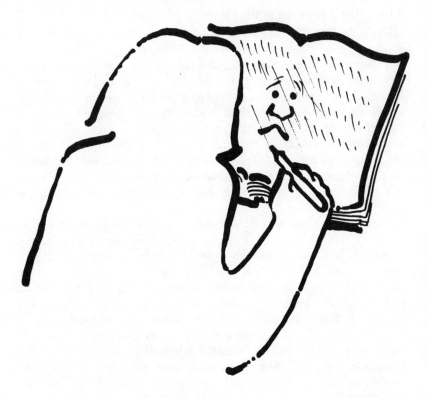

The feelings we record in a journal can act as a verbal mirror, reflecting back our attitudes and opinions.

letting the boss make you eat like that." Another, more constructive and self-sustaining opinion is: "My reaction to the tension I experienced at work (overeating) is not a constructive way of dealing with my feelings, because it makes me feel worse about myself. A better way to deal with my feelings is to _____."
Fill in the blank: "take a long walk"? "play the guitar, which I'm good at and which always reminds me that I like myself"? The latter response is also an opinion of sorts. But it is primarily an observation, coupled with a positive judgment about a behavior that would work for you.

Okay, let's give it a go. Begin, right now, by opening your notebook to the first page.

First, mark today's date and the time.

Next, write a brief account of what went on in your day and how you feel about it.

Now, recount, *factually and dispassionately,* your eating behavior for the day:" At 8:00 A.M., I ate a scrambled egg. At 9:00 A.M., I ate the kids' leftover toast and jam." And so forth.

Next, write several sentences (at least four) that begin with the words "I feel":

I FEEL _____

I FEEL _____

I FEEL _____

I FEEL _____

You can use the blank spaces above to record what you feel at this moment. Just let it flow — don't think, DO! Freudians call this "free association," William James called it "stream of consciousness," and I call it "letting go and letting it flow." HOW DO YOU FEEL? In journal-reporting like this, it is imperative that you take the passion out. Reporting your feelings and forming judgments about them are two entirely different things. One says, "I feel disappointed in my behavior *in this instance,*" while the other says, "My behavior just goes to show what an awful person I am." Do not focus on what you hate or love about your behavior. Merely report it. And use the word *choose.* For example, you could write, "I ate like a pig today because Sally and I went to lunch together and she insisted that I eat more than I wanted and I feel like a fat slob." That's a good example of a self-negating report. After all, did Sally force you to eat the Linguini Alfredo rather than the Salada Fresca? Your journal entry would be more realistic and more self-supporting if you were to write: "I *chose* to have lunch with Sally today, knowing her effect on me where food is concerned. I *chose* to overeat. I *feel* that it is more difficult to make a constructive choice when I eat with Sally. When she prompts me to eat in ways that conflict with my goal for desired weight, it is more difficult to eat in control. I may *choose* to have lunch with a more supportive person next time."

The phrase "next time" needs to appear at the end of every journal entry. After reviewing the day's events, your "I feel" lines, and your observations about what you chose to do during the day, add at least four "next time" lines:

NEXT TIME, I will _____

NEXT TIME, I would feel better if _____

NEXT TIME, I choose to _____

NEXT TIME, _____

To sum up, there are five basic steps to follow in your daily journal-writing:

(1) Write the date and time of day.

(2) Write a brief account of your day and your feelings about it.

(3) Write what your eating behavior was during the day.

(4) Write at least four "I feel" lines.

(5) Write at least four "next time" lines.

Because, for most of us, it is difficult to write our observations and feelings without injecting self-damaging judgments, it is often useful to write two drafts of every journal entry at first. The rough draft will allow you to "let go and let it flow"; the second, final draft, to be written by editing the first draft on the morning following the reported day's events, will allow you to practice your objective, nonjudgmental reporting skills (and will remind you of how you felt the day before if you overate). After a few such revisions, you will become more adept at simply observing your behavior, without either condemning it or praising it.

DOs AND DON'Ts: SAMPLE ENTRIES

Here are three examples of what not to do and what to do when writing your journal entries. Each pair represents an actual entry that went through revision as the writer, whom I'll call Amy, learned the difference between judging and simply noticing her behavior.

Example 1

What Not To Do:
4/23, 8:00 P.M. Today was a drag. If this house doesn't sell soon, I'll go crazy. Tom yelled about the dog again today. Let him get rid of the dog — I'm not going to. Naturally, after the dog incident I ate like a pig. Every damned time Tom blows up, I just eat like it's going out of style. Also, the house just sits here while the realtor drags her feet, so of course I got mad and ate a ton. I'm not saying what I ate, I just ate, that's all.

I FEEL like hell.

I FEEL frustrated.

I FEEL disappointed in myself.

I FEEL like crying — I am crying!

NEXT TIME I don't know what to say.

NEXT TIME I'll do better.

NEXT TIME I'll tell Tom to go to hell — just kidding!

NEXT TIME — No, I wasn't kidding, he can take the dog back — *I'm* not going to!

What To Do:
4/23, 8:00 P.M. Today could have been better. I get so bored sitting here waiting for this house to sell. When Tom yelled at me to get rid of the dog so the yard would look better for the house sale, I got furious. Actually, I got hurt, too. I sit here all day waiting for the real estate lady, who doesn't show up, and I'm the one picking up the dog poop!

I *chose* to eat after Tom yelled at me. It is a hard pattern for me to break. I'm so used to doing it. Also, when 6:00 P.M. rolled around and not one person had come to look at the house, I ate all of the leftover dinner rolls from last night.

I FEEL burdened by the house.

I FEEL angry and disappointed that Tom yelled at me.

I FEEL sad that I did that to myself (ate the rolls).

I FEEL that I let myself down.

NEXT TIME I'm telling Tom how I feel — I get frustrated, too.

NEXT TIME I'm waiting only until 3:00 P.M., and then I'm leaving.

NEXT TIME I will go for a long walk or get on the rebounder when I'm angry before I choose whether to eat.

NEXT TIME I'll throw the rolls away the night before!

Notice the difference between Amy's two drafts. She brought the first draft in and we reworked it until she got the idea of how to do it. The first draft was much too general, for one thing. What does it mean, "Today was a drag"? Be specific. The second time, Amy was specific: She was bored and frustrated that the house wasn't selling and that she was stuck there until six in the evening. She was angry and hurt that Tom yelled about the dog, adding to her frustration.

The "I feel" lines are where you can really let your feelings out — not in generalities, but in specific terms. Notice that "I feel like hell" (in Amy's first draft) neither defines her emotion nor explains *why* she was feeling that way. With "disappointed" and "frustrated," she got closer, but she still needed to pinpoint the "why." She does so in her second draft, simply stating the source of the emotion — "burdened by the house," for example.

The "next time" lines are intended to help you build a better plan. It is obvious in the first draft that Amy hadn't given that much thought. She went from saying she didn't know what to do next time to experiencing tears. In her second draft, she began to plan ahead, listing what she would do under similar circumstances.

Example 2

What Not To Do:

5/1, 9:00 P.M. Well, today was rather dull. Nothing much happened. The guy came about the fence and botched it up good. I told Tom he ought to get a real fence guy, not a "handyman," but no, not Tom. Boring day.

My eating was not lousy but not good either. I did manage to stay under control until that idiot messed up the fence. That was it — I hit the potato chips!

I FEEL blah — you know, just blah.

I FEEL tired of it all. (Sounds morbid, huh?)

I FEEL like running away. (Where?)

I FEEL really angry when Tom is so cheap. What's the saying — "pennywise and pound foolish"? That's him, all right.

NEXT TIME I know I'm supposed to say I'll do better, but will I?

NEXT TIME I'll send the guy home and call the fence man myself.

NEXT TIME I will run away. (Not really!)

NEXT TIME I'll fix the damned fence myself! Less anguish that way.

What To Do:
5/1, 9:00 P.M. I was bored today from feeling compelled to SIT in this house and wait for the fence man. I am very angry that Tom insists on trying to cut corners and hire some kid to fix it. It is in terrible shape. I'm also angry that I had to keep the dog in the basement while that kid supposedly fixed the fence.

My eating reflected my anger, no doubt about it. After writing here for only one week, it's becoming clear. I ate lightly all morning and afternoon until that kid came to "fix" the fence. When he left, I ate the rest of the potato chips and other leftovers, and even finished off the oatmeal from breakfast. Oh well, no judgments, right? Hard not to make me wrong, but I guess I did what I did and it's done. Finished, over with, "spilt oatmeal."

I FEEL unable to communicate my feelings to Tom directly.

I FEEL uneasy about telling him how cheap he is (but he really is).

I FEEL that this whole fence thing would move quicker if I took charge.

I FEEL I'd best get busy and take that assertiveness-training class in the spring.

NEXT TIME I'll at least tell Tom that I'm frustrated that I can't communicate with him.

NEXT TIME I'll *suggest* that I handle the fence and see how that flies.

NEXT TIME I'll take the dog for a long walk in the park when the fence man is here.

NEXT TIME I really will say *something* to Tom so I will quit swallowing my anger — and that yucky oatmeal (should've tossed it after breakfast). Funny that I never noticed before how often I eat when I'm angry.

We can begin to see how Amy has progressed in only one week. The first draft is still full of complaints that aren't clearly spelled out, but it's better than her previous week's report. In the second draft, she has become much clearer about her need to enhance her communication with Tom. The first "I feel" lines were vague, but the second time around it was clear what her true feelings were. She even pinpointed how she was swallowing her anger.

The second draft also reflects a better plan for improvement in the "next time" section. In the first draft, Amy wanted only to escape; with the second, she is willing to take an assertiveness-training class to learn to cope rather than escape. Great progress for her!

Example 3

What Not To Do:

5/10, 8:45 P.M. Today I had a pleasant day away from the house for a change. Mary and I went shopping. Still, I find it hard to shop when she buys a size 12 dress and I'm looking through the size 16s — again. I get real envious feelings, even though I love her dearly. Sometimes she's not very thoughtful when she prances around asking me if the dress is too tight, etc. I never find anything that looks good on me — just more of the same old stuff in stripes!

I did real well with food while with Mary. She had a tuna salad sandwich and I just had the tuna salad. I felt good about that. But when I came home, I thought about the cruddy-looking clothes and felt bad. When Tom asked me why I hadn't bought something and not just wasted my time running from store to store, I got teed off. After Tom went to bed, I ate the last of the kids' chocolate bars and hid the wrappers at the bottom of the trash can. I can't believe I did that, but I did. If anyone finds this journal, I'll croak!

I FEEL good to get out of the house.

I FEEL pretty sick about the clothing selection in my size.

I FEEL that Mary can be thoughtless about my feelings.

I FEEL like never shopping again.

NEXT TIME I'll just watch her shop and I'll stop looking.

NEXT TIME I'll shop with someone as fat as I am.

NEXT TIME I'll complain to the store manager about the lousy selection.

NEXT TIME I'll forget shopping!

What To Do:
5/10, 8:45 P.M. Today it was great to be away from the house. Mary and I went shopping. I found myself feeling envious of her cute figure. I felt rather angry when she asked two or three times if that dynamite size 12 dress was too skimpy or too tight. It seemed like she was wanting me to notice that she fits a size 12 perfectly. I felt like telling her she looked great, already — enough! I hereby resolve to stop shopping until I get to at least a size 14. I am agonizing over having to wear a size 16, and it's not worth it.

My eating was in control with Mary. I had a tuna salad and iced tea, but I let it get out of control after Tom asked why I hadn't bought anything and said that I had wasted my time. It is too complicated (or maybe it is too embarrassing) to tell him why I didn't buy something. So I ate out of control after Tom went to bed. That tells me a lot. Again with the unexpressed anger, already. I have the catalog from the community college and I am enrolling in the assertiveness-training class for sure. I can use it.

I FEEL that I need to learn to express to Mary how embarrassing it is for me when she continually asks me how good she looks.

I FEEL angry when she fishes for compliments.

I FEEL humiliated when Tom seems disappointed that I didn't buy something.

I FEEL like nobody knows how horrible shopping is for a fat person!

NEXT TIME I'll say something to Mary (after I take the class, ha!).

NEXT TIME I'll level with Tom and tell him how sad I feel looking at clothes.

NEXT TIME I'll resolve that *for now* I have a small selection, but soon I will be able to shop like a real human being.

NEXT TIME I won't have to eat the chocolate bars when Tom is asleep if I tell him the truth. He doesn't even have a clue how horrible it is for me to be humiliated in a department store. He needs to know, and I need to be able to tell him without feeling embarrassed.

In these three examples, we see real progress in Amy's attitudes. The second draft of this last example is more definite than the first two examples, and the "next time" lines are more future-oriented. This third entry is much more expressive of Amy's true feelings. Even the first draft is far superior to what she wrote two weeks before, when she was putting herself down. She still judges herself — right for "good" behavior (tuna salad) and wrong for "bad" behavior (chocolate bars) — but she's not totally down on herself. She can't believe she ate the chocolate bars, but there are no more bad names.

The general level of Amy's insight is increasing. She now sees the need to express herself more fully to both Tom and Mary. She is beginning to see that her lack of full self-expression has hindered her throughout her life.

In the second draft, in the "I feel" lines, Amy is more honest about her deeply hurt emotions. She is willing to commit them to paper, and she even considers sharing them with her husband. She has gained the insight that he doesn't have a "clue" how horrifying it is for her to shop and find nothing. She feels humiliated and used by Mary's fishing for compliments and her subtle, covert comparisons of the two women's bodies.

Amy is on the move now, and she's growing daily. She has neared her desired weight, she has sold the house, and she has taken the assertiveness-training class. She has kept her weight at a steady 132 pounds for two years and, although she still feels that 125 is her desired weight, she is pleased with her plateau and feels that with further involvement in school and other outlets for self-expression, the additional pounds will come off. She wears a size 12 and sometimes a 10 (eat your heart out, Mary!) and feels confident that she'll never shop at Omar the Tent-Maker's again!

WRITE ON

Remember that you can control your old faulty food tapes —both your early childhood tapes and your current social tapes. Your journal-writing is essential to breaking into these tapes and helping you to redirect your thinking in non-food-focused ways.

Keeping your journal for at least six weeks will facilitate your left-brain awareness of the highly subjective right-brain experiences you are about to undergo as you work through the next two chapters. In fact, I recommend that you continue keeping your journal as you add the more advanced Reflective Relearning exercises in which you are about to engage. Combining the left-brain (journal) exercises with the right-brain Reflective Relearning program will give you a strong base from which to build a new relationship with food, as the two sides of the brain and the two functions of the mind learn to work in tandem.

As you progress through the six weeks of journal-writing and then add the six-week Reflective Relearning program described in Chapter 8, you will increase your skill in separating negative self-judgment from dispassionate observation, which will make new learning possible. It is difficult to learn new habits when old experiences and behavior patterns block the way.

As you will learn in the next chapter, you can willfully induce and direct your own normally occurring altered states of consciousness by using your left brain and conscious mind to tap into the highly influential right brain and subconscious mind. When you do this, you are allowing your intuitive right brain to begin moving toward altering your eating behavior *as you choose.*

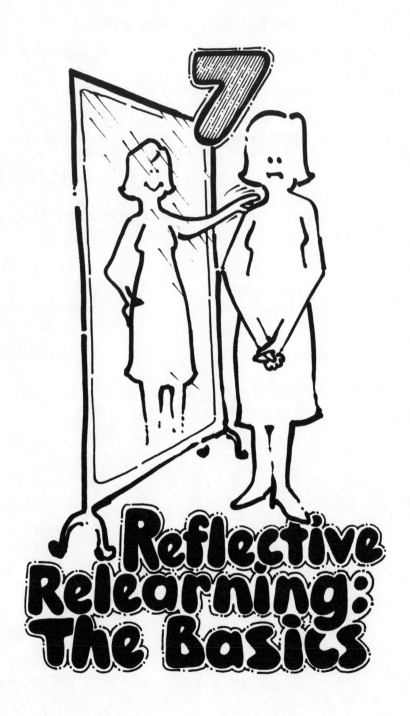

Reflective Relearning: The Basics

YOU HAVE LEARNED FROM THE PREVIOUS CHAPTER the insights that may be gained through journal-writing. This process allows your left-brain, conscious side to feel a sense of control while simultaneously allowing the intuitive right brain to start expressing its insights. The next step is to learn to allow your right-brain images and subconscious thoughts to manifest themselves with minimal intervention by the left brain. This step is very important because it goes far beyond the left-brain processes called upon by journal-writing. For the first time, you will learn how to know the "hidden" thoughts, emotions, and attitudes that journal-writing cannot reveal in depth. Now we are moving to another dimension of awareness, which functions very differently from the conscious, logical mind.

This kind of awareness involves being receptive, silent and calm, like a still pool of water, to allow right brain images to surface as clearly as possible. I call this a state of *Reflection*. The actual process of taking this insight into our left brain "conscious" awareness and using it to change old, habitual responses is called reprogramming, or *Relearning*. Hence the term I have used a few times before now, and will be using a great deal in the next two chapters — Reflective Relearning. Reflective Relearning is an essential step in taking control of your eating behavior. Whereas journal-writing opened the door for investigation, Reflective Relearning opens the windows wide for you to get a fuller view of what you need to DO in order to obtain, maintain, and sustain your desired weight. In this chapter, then, we will begin to do just that — throw open the windows for a wider vista of YOU.

ALTERED STATES OF CONSCIOUSNESS:
THE PATH TO THE RIGHT BRAIN
AND THE SUBCONSCIOUS MIND

First, let's talk about normally occurring altered states of consciousness. How do you and I alter our "normal" state of consciousness? We dream, we daydream, we have states of fragmentation (ever open a drawer and wonder what in the world it was you were looking for? — that's fragmentation). There is the state of half-waking half-sleeping, called "hypnagogic" when we are going to sleep, and "hypnopompic" when we are coming out of sleep. These are all altered states of consciousness, and they occur normally, unlike those induced by drugs.

In other words, these normal states of altered consciousness occur nearly every day of our lives, even though we are usually unaware of them. It seems as if almost everything has to lie within our left-brain, conscious, verbal, logical awareness for us to know it. When the subconscious mind wants to get some message across, the left brain, conscious part of us keeps refusing to "get the picture." Perhaps our right-brain, subconscious dreams have been telling us for a long time that there's something we need to attend to, but the left-brain, logical side dismisses it as mere "fantasy." After enough such dismissals, the subconscious mind may send something that really gets our attention, like a terrifying nightmare. Now we begin to listen! The right brain has made contact with the left brain; the subconscious has become conscious.

There are many safe ways to place ourselves purposefully in these normally occurring altered states of consciousness. That is, we can make a conscious decision to allow ourselves to phase into these states of awareness, where we are more receptive to our subconscious messages. Once we get our right brain and left brain "talking" in this way, we can begin to reprogram our thinking patterns. If in the past you and I have subconsciously linked food, security and comfort together, we can now de-link and reassociate these feelings with other thinking levels. Some psychologists call this process hypnosis or self-hypnosis. As you know, I call it Reflective Relearning.

HYPNOTHERAPY: DEPTH
OF FOCUS OR HOCUS-POCUS?

I often ask people if they have ever been hypnotized. Usually, they say they have not. Some even say they went to a hypnotist and the hypnosis didn't "take." The truth is, most people don't understand what the hypnotic state really is. They typically conjure up pictures of an evil-looking man swinging a pocket watch in front of someone, telling that person to "relax, relax, relax." Then they envision the "victim" falling into some deep, stuporlike trance, completely at the will of the hypnotist, and clucking like a chicken or doing some other foolish thing.

This common picture of hypnosis is, to say the least, inaccurate. In fact, while they are under hypnosis (either self-hypnosis or other-directed hypnosis), most people remain quite aware of what is happening around them. Hypnosis is properly defined as a "heightened state of awareness." That is, we are *more* rather than *less* aware of what is going on. Furthermore, in the hypnotic state of consciousness our awareness level is channeled into a narrow band of attention. We "hone in" on whatever it is that interests us, either with self-direction or under the direction of the hypnotherapist.

Another popular misconception about hypnosis is that it is a sleeping state. Hypnosis can lead to a sleeping state, but if a person under hypnosis falls asleep, he is no longer hypnotized — he is simply asleep. Some people express the fear that they might "go under" so deeply that they will never emerge from the hypnotic state. There is no such thing as "going under" in this sense — only sleep, if it occurs at all.

Some people confuse hypnotherapy with brainwashing, like in the Svengali-Trilby story, in which the innocent subject is victimized. They think of hypnosis as a devious technique by which the therapist can impose his or her will on them, and coerce them into accepting a different value system, regardless of how they feel about those values.

Let me give you an example of the difference between hypnosis and brainwashing. If someone were to come to me to be hypnotized, and he trusted me, he would probably follow my suggestions. If I were to ask him to sing a song under hypnosis, he probably would, because singing is something he is likely to do in front of someone, at least once in a while anyway. Likewise, if I asked him to do a little dance while hypnotized, he might be likely to dance, too. Now, let me show you how hypnosis can be misused. If I were to ask a hypnotized person to take his clothes off in front of me, he would not, unless he were an exhibitionist or a nudist. However, if I wished to mislead this person, I might suggest that he is preparing for a shower, and should remove his clothing and step into the shower. This is how brainwashing is accomplished. A charlatan *could* mislead someone into taking his clothes off, and the hypnotized person would follow directions, because he would actually believe he was about to take a shower.

If you are thinking about having another person guide you into an altered state, then it is mandatory that you get the names of licensed hypnotherapists. You should also be aware that there is a difference between a hypnotist and a hypnotherapist. Not that one necessarily does the process better than the other, but the licensed practitioner — the hypnotherapist — has valid training which you can check.

STAYING IN YOUR RIGHT MIND ·

Hypnosis, then (or self-hypnosis, depending on who is leading the process), is simply a heightened state of awareness in a narrow band of attention. Many people, after they find out what the hypnotic state really is, are amazed to find that they have indeed been in a self-hypnotic state many times. For example, have you ever driven down the road, blissfully happy — only to find yourself three turnoffs past your intended exit? Why did this happen? Where were you? Your body was there driving the car, but where were *you?* Your thoughts were obviously elsewhere. You see, when I'm driving down the highway and having a wonderful romantic conversation with Robert Redford, I'm not very concerned with the signs. What usually happens is that I stay in my fantasy and miss my exit. Of course, if another car were to swerve into my lane, Robert would fly right out the window and I would jump back into my body and *be there.* You see, when the conscious mind is needed, it is readily available. But when what's going on is mundane, repetitive — boring — the conscious mind tends to slow down and lose interest.

One of the main functions of our left brain and conscious

mind is figuring things out. When there's nothing for the left brain to figure out, it tends to disengage. The subconscious, right-brain, emotional side of us tends to take over then. A much-needed balancing between the conscious and subconscious minds and the left and right cerebral hemispheres continually takes place through our normal altered states of consciousness.

There is nothing occult or mysterious about sitting quietly and reflecting upon what you want your body to look like. We are simply getting to know our subconscious mind and right brain — learning to "talk" to it. We can begin to repeat to ourselves that, instead of eating, we will (for example) take a quiet walk for half an hour in order to feel better. After a few weeks, this message becomes absorbed by the subconscious mind. Your wonderful right brain helps you further the process by allowing you to picture yourself actually walking instead of eating.

I realize that there are skeptics who will dismiss this as the same "positive thinking stuff" that has been around for years. Yes, it is positive thinking. The difference, however, is that as of the last fifteen or twenty years, we have been gathering scientific, empirical evidence that shows why it works. It doesn't work through some magical process; it works because of the functioning of the right brain and the subconscious mind. You and I must constantly remind ourselves that, although it feels like the reality the conscious mind shows us is the only one there is, our right brain and subconscious mind — our subtle, silent partners —also have a very distinct reality.

Sometimes I'll ask a client, "Do you ever talk to yourself?" The answer is invariably an emphatic yes. We *all* talk to ourselves, almost all the time, even when we're in altered states such as dreaming or daydreaming. This self-talk is the way the thought process occurs. Occasionally, we find ourselves talking aloud to ourselves. This usually happens when we are in deep concentration, when we are totally focused on one channel of thought. There is a phenomenon called "completion of the language loop." It means that sometimes, when we are deeply involved in one line of thought, we like to hear the words come out of our mouths and into our ears. It's like a double reinforcement. It makes what we are focusing on even clearer.

Since we all constantly talk to ourselves (the real question is do we ever shut up!), we need to be able to attend to some of this self-dialogue. One way to do this is simply to become conscious of having a daydream. Then we can decide if this is a line of thought we consciously want to follow. For example, you notice that you are in your car driving home from work, mumbling about what might be in the refrigerator. The moment you become consciously aware of where these random, subconsciously driven thoughts are leading you, you may decide, consciously, to intervene. You can stop focusing on the refrigerator and say out loud, "Wait, let me think about taking a walk first; then I'll explore eating possibilities." Such relearning is crucial for each of us. We have to reprogram our thinking patterns.

This new kind of talking to ourselves sometimes seems too simple to be valid. Yet some of the most powerful things in the world are simple. The left-brain, logical side of you and me will want to dismiss all this as a waste of time. But I can assure you that taking time to become conscious of our thought processes is worth every minute. I sometimes jokingly tell people to "stay in their bodies" as much as possible. By this I mean, *become aware of what you are doing at the time you are doing it.* You see, we spend a great deal of time thinking about what we might have said in the past, or what we will do about some future event. We spend very little time in the here-and-now.

It is important to take stock of what you're dwelling on when you're "lost in thought," and consciously to bring yourself back to earth. Bringing ourselves to the here-and-now and focusing on what is happening in our thought patterns allows us to make conscious decisions: Do I want to continue this chain of thought or switch to a more productive one? When I notice my right brain forming images of food while I'm watching television, triggering my subconscious mind to put forth the old "eat" tapes, I can switch to planning what color size 9 dress to buy for that special occasion next month.

This simple procedure of "staying in your right mind" is difficult at first, because it seems foreign to us to listen to our thoughts. Many, many thoughts pass through our minds every minute. And for those of us who have learned to solve our problems by reaching for food, many of those thoughts are reflecting this very process of faulty problem solving. That's why it is imperative to interrupt the flow of food thoughts and replace it with thinking patterns that promote wellness and help you to obtain, maintain, and sustain your desired weight for life.

THE ABCs OF REFLECTIVE RELEARNING

We come now to the basic of Reflective Relearning, or R&R, as I sometimes like to call it, because Reflective Relearning not only helps us get in touch with ourselves and reach our goals, it also provides the "rest and relaxation" — the real stress release — that too many of us have replaced with overeating.

In the remainder of this chapter, I will outline the basic procedures involved in this simple yet powerful method of keeping ourselves in touch with our right-brain perceptions and subconscious thoughts. This introduction to the "building block," the basic ten-minute Reflective Relearning session, will prepare you to undertake the step-by-step six-week program presented in Chapter 8. In those weekly sessions you will find different relaxation techniques to use before you come to the basic Reflective Relearning affirmation presented here. As you approach your desired weight, you may wish to modify the basic affirmation to help you meet life goals other than weight management.

Starting Out

The first thing you need to do is set aside a time and a place for this self-reflection. It is imperative that you allow yourself *ten minutes per day devoted exclusively to you.* Ten minutes a day of QUALITY time spent alone amounts to 3,650 minutes per year, or about 68 hours, or not quite three full days of 24 hours each. That's not much to ask, yet that is all you need to tap the tremendous power within you through Reflective Relearning.

By the way, this time by yourself, when you reflect quietly on how you wish to be, does not conflict with any religious belief. It's like comparing apples and shoes — there's not much of a connection! The word "meditate" means "to focus one's thoughts on, reflect or ponder on; to plan or project in the mind." Synonyms for meditation include "intent" and "purpose," and a further definition states that meditation is "to engage in contemplation or reflection." When I use the term "Reflective Relearning," this is the tone I wish to impart. If you happen to be a religious person, you may choose to combine this time with prayerful activity. You do not, however, need to have a religious orientation for Reflective Relearning to work for you. Just remember that there are certain universal truths, and one of them is that life progresses from thought to action to form. In Reflective Relearning, we work with the thought that leads to the form.

Once you have *decided* to allow yourself ten minutes every day to reflect on your eating behavior and to relearn that behavior, you need to choose the specific time of the day when you will engage in this meditative process. Choose a time that you can stick with — one when you are least likely to be disturbed or face outside pressures. Some people find it best to set aside ten minutes in the morning, when they are fresh. Others prefer the evening, when the concerns of work and family have receded for the day. The particular time of day you choose is less important than the regularity of it; doing your exercises at the same time of day, every day, will make "getting into the habit" much faster and easier.

More difficult than finding the daily ten minutes (everyone can spare ten minutes a day) or a regular time of day is finding a place where you can unplug the phone and hang out your "do not disturb" sign. When I first began doing this process for myself (and, by the way, I still do it for at least ten minutes a day and usually longer), I used my walk-in closet. I had three active young boys and there was lots of commotion going on around me all day. I chose to do my Reflective Relearning first thing in the morning, when the children were usually asleep. As they grew up, their schedules changed, since they are swimmers and go to workouts as early as 5:30 A.M. So I had to be sure to put out my sign and get into my closet fast!

Some people with whom I have worked have found ingenious ways to be alone. One woman who works for a huge law firm

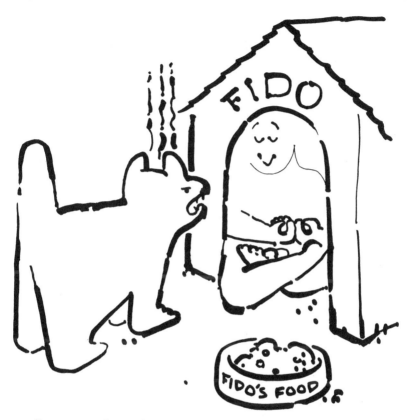

**Some people with whom I have worked have found
ingenious ways to be alone.**

simply goes down to the parking lot and sits in her car for ten
minutes every day during her coffee break. A young mother I
know has a high school girl drop by on her way home from
school daily for twenty minutes while Mom drives to a nearby
quiet park and does her Reflective Relearning there. There's
always a way to find the time and the place — the idea is to
FIND THEM! Do not let yourself down — you owe it to you.

Okay, so here you are, in your chosen place. You're ready to
begin. It's important to wear loose clothing and sit in a cool spot

where it's not so warm that you're likely to drift into sleep.

It would be helpful for you to review Chapter 1 at this point. As you begin to do this process, I want you to appreciate intellectually what the functions of the right and left brain are, as well as the workings of the conscious and subconscious mind. After the review, you will remember that one of the first challenges for anyone doing Reflective Relearning is to put the left brain at ease. The left cerebral hemisphere truly believes that if it loses control, everything will fall apart. Therefore, you must be able to acknowledge the left, verbal, rational side of your brain at all times. Even when you are deeply relaxed and stating your goal over and over, the left side will suddenly pop up and tell you to let the cat out (or something like that). When this happens — and it will happen over and over again — simply remark to yourself, "Yes, thank you. I will attend to the cat later. Now I consciously choose to return to my Reflective Relearning process." At the beginning, this is the biggest hurdle for most people to get over. People ask me, "When will these thoughts stop popping into my head?" The answer is, "Maybe never." The important thing to focus on is the rapidity with which you make a conscious choice to return to your Reflective Relearning state.

Sometimes, when you first sit down to be still, it is useful to imagine that there is a knob on each side of your head. These are your volume-control knobs, and you can imagine yourself turning the volume on the left side down as you simultaneously turn the volume on the right side up. This can also help set the mood for your session. Yet, be aware that from time to time your left side will continue to feed you information, and this information may be vital, so it is important that you acknowledge it. After all, if your verbal side yells "SMOKE! — Get out of here!" you want to hear that! Usually, the left side will feed you mundane, repetitious information that you should feel free to dismiss. Occasionally, however, it is important to listen. So don't turn the left side off, just turn it down.

Okay, you've reminded yourself intellectually of what you can expect from your left brain as you embark on this process. You are alone in your chosen spot — quiet and ready to begin.

Relaxing and Focusing

For the first minute or so, simply sit in a comfortable position — preferably in a straight-backed chair with arms (so you don't sway when your body is relaxed) — and breathe deeply. As you inhale slowly and deeply, repeat to yourself
I AM,
and as you exhale deeply and slowly, repeat to yourself
RELAXED.
Do this for about a minute. If you are breathing very deeply and very slowly, you should do about four rounds in one minute. It is best to breathe through your nostrils if you can do so comfortably.

Sitting in your chair, be sure both feet are flat on the floor and your hands are resting in your lap or by your sides, preferably with the palms up. When we turn our palms downward, we tend unconsciously to grasp, and this can be a source of distraction. You may also choose to sit on the floor. If you use a chair, be sure it supports the small of your back, or use a small, firm pillow for lower back support. Soft, fluffy chairs are a poor choice, because your back will eventually tire. Sometimes when I sit in a chair for my own Reflective Relearning exercises, I roll up a small hand towel and place it at the small of my back for comfort and support.

Now, for the next minute or so, allow your breathing to return to normal and simply listen to your thoughts as they flow by. Pay close attention to your rational, busy left brain. It will send you many messages per second. It will remind you to get milk when you go to the store. It will admonish you for sitting here doing "nothing." The left cerebral hemisphere always wants to figure things out, and when you sit quietly there isn't much to figure out, so it becomes alarmed and restless. Nevertheless, allow your left brain and conscious thoughts to wander, and watch your thoughts as if your were viewing a television screen. Acknowledge each thought and let it pass right on by.

For the next minute or so, simply tune in to any sounds around you. Focus on any distractions. You may hear the hum of the refrigerator, a bird, a dog barking, or a car passing by. Listen very carefully for these sounds and make a mental note of them.

About three minutes have elapsed since you sat down. Now begin to repeat to yourself silently:

I NOW MAKE A CONSCIOUS DECISION TO RELEASE ALL SOUNDS AROUND ME.

Say this to yourself three or four times. Then make the following statement to yourself silently at least three times:

I NOW CONSCIOUSLY ALLOW MYSELF TO LET ALL THOUGHTS AND SOUNDS FALL AWAY.

Now spend another minute imagining that you are staring into a blank screen. As thoughts come to you, consciously dismiss them and return to staring into your blank screen. Approximately five minutes have now passed since you sat down. You are ready for phase two, the actual reprogramming.

Choosing a Goal

Let's backtrack now for a moment. I was so anxious to get you started, we didn't even talk about choosing the goal that you will work towards. How you define and state your goal is very, very important, and there are certain rules you should follow. Your goal should be in your mind before you sit down. Your goal must be stated positively. If necessary, write it out before you start until you get the "hang" of it. A positive goal is one that is both specific and reasonable. A goal statement such as "I want to be skinny" is not specific enough; it is also potentially dangerous. The subconscious mind may pick up the suggestion and you may become too thin. I know it doesn't seem that way now, but it can happen — and has been known to happen among anorexics. If you want to work on an improved lifestyle, be sure you are specific about that too. The goal statement "I want to be happy" is too vague. A more specific goal statement would be, "I see myself sharing loving, quality time with my husband and children."

Some goals may seem positive yet are negative in how they are expressed. "I will no longer bite my fingernails," for example, is not a positive goal. You can rephrase it this way:" I see my fingernails as long, strong and beautiful." If you are using this time to control smoking, you would set the goal: "I see myself as a happy, healthy nonsmoker."

Now, you may ask, "What is a reasonable amount of time for me to gain my desired weight?" Depending upon your nutritional program, you can move toward your goal by one or two pounds per week. This is a reasonable amount of weight to change during a week, and not too much. It has been proven nutritionally that when people drop weight too rapidly, the body sends out messages that all fat must be stored. It's afraid of starvation. If you were lost in the Andes, you would be glad you have this survival mechanism!

One goal for weight management that has proved to be especially valuable for those using it is this:

"I WILL ALLOW MYSELF TO OBTAIN, MAINTAIN, AND SUSTAIN MY DESIRED WEIGHT OF_____ POUNDS (Insert your desired weight here, and be sure you can see this numeral with your mind's eye) BY_____ ."
(Insert a reasonable date — say, six months down the line if you wish to shed fifty pounds — and don't forget the year; be sure you also see this date with your mind's eye.)

Remember, we all visualize differently. If you're having trouble "seeing" the weight numeral and the date clearly, imagine that you are standing in front of a large chalkboard with a large piece of chalk in your hand. Imagine yourself writing the weight and the date over and over again.

Another way to "see" with your mind's eye is to write your desired weight and date on a large piece of unlined white paper with a black grease pen. Stare at this for a while and then close your eyes. You will probably see the "negative" of what you wrote — that is, you will see white numerals on a black background.

Some people never literally "see" their weight written out. They merely get some visual impressions. That's fine. You don't need to see real numerals before you. People who report never being able to visualize literally still have marvelous results.

A very common question people ask is how to keep track of time when they are reflecting with their eyes closed. At the beginning, it is best to have a digital clock or watch handy. (Do not use a timer with a bell or a buzzer. The sudden sound will jar you into a state of alarm and ruin your relaxation.) The first phase, deep breathing, usually consists of about four long, deep inhalations and exhalations — about one minute. Time yourself at the beginning to see how many rounds you do in one minute. The next phase, allowing the left-brain, rational part of your awareness to roam freely and listening consciously for outside sounds, also takes about one minute (or perhaps a minute and a half). It's okay to open your eyes occasionally to check the lapsed time. Eventually your subconscious mind will know exactly how much time has passed during each phase, and your timepiece will become unnecessary.

As you can see, the first half of your process is basically a technique to allow your left brain to still itself while the right, visual side begins to be stimulated. Staring into the blank screen of your mind's eye is an excellent way to still the left cerebral hemisphere and ready the right, visual side for action. During the actual reprogramming phase, when you repeat your goal to yourself for three or four minutes, your right brain will come into action as you visualize your desired weight and the date written out before your eyes. Later on, you may want to change this goal to actually see yourself in a mirror the way you desire to be.

Now let's assume that you have gone through the entire process. Here's a recap:

(1) Sit for about one minute and breathe deeply, repeating "I AM RELAXED" — "I am" on the inhalation, and "relaxed" on the exhalation.

(2) Spend the next minute or so allowing your left brain to scan and feed information to you. Let it tell you everything it has to say for a minute or so.

(3) Spend the next minute or so consciously listening to your environment, picking up sounds and making mental notes by focusing on them.

(4) For the next minute or so, make conscious statements to yourself about your conscious intent to let all sounds fall away, as you are now ready to enter phase two of your Reflective Relearning state.

(5) Now is the time of the actual reprogramming. State your positive goal to yourself in no more than fifteen words. Keep repeating this goal for at least three minutes.

(6) As you prepare to return to your normal state of consciousness, give yourself one positive statement which will help you carry this goal through the rest of your day. You may say, "I fully intend to reach my goal" as you move from your relaxed state to your normal awareness state.

(7) At the end of the ten minutes, gradually begin to wiggle your fingers and toes and stretch your body. Open your eyes and return to your normal state of awareness.

Naturally, as you practice this technique, you will become relaxed and receptive in progressively shorter spans of time. I now spend only a minute in totally releasing and relaxing instead of the three to five minutes I spent fifteen years ago, when I first began. Give yourself time to feel comfortable with the process.

FORM THE HABIT

At this point, you have two specific things to do in order to put it all together. First, be faithful to the four-step journal-writing method of Chapter 6. Second, be faithful to the basic ten-minute Reflective Relearning technique presented in this chapter. Make these techniques a habit — a part of your daily ritual of self-care, as important as grooming and (yes!) eating healthy, well-balanced, well-sized meals.

To help you get into the daily habit of Reflective Relearning, and replace the faulty problem-solving habit of overeating, the next chapter outlines a six-week program of Reflective Relearning sessions designed especially for those new to the practice. Follow this regimen faithfully through the full forty-two days, and you will get into the habit of Reflective Relearning — a *positive* habit that will gradually but surely replace the negative pain chain of overeating that could keep you from being and getting the best in life. Read on — and be prepared for amazing results as you move toward taking control of your eating for life.

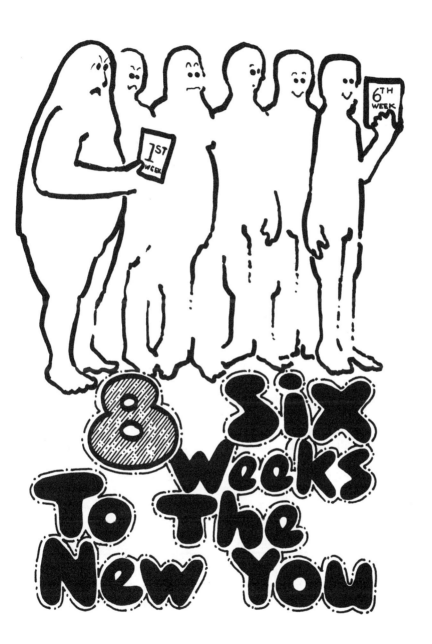

IF YOU'VE COME THIS FAR, you've come a long way, baby! You are now keeping a journal on your attitudes toward your eating behavior (to satisfy the good ol' left brain), and you've tried the basic Reflective Relearning (R&R) technique outlined in Chapter 7, at least once. So now everything's hunky-dory, right?

No? You mean you're still hitting that goodie-filled fridge at the first sign of stress? Well, despair not. In this instant-gratification society, it's no surprise that many of us return to old, comforting habits if a new technique doesn't work the first time out. That's why you've come to this chapter, because you and I both know that it takes time and self-discipline to form new habits. And that's why, in this chapter, I intend to make it easier for you to do just that, by outlining a six-week plan of Reflective Relearning exercises that will quiet down your busybody left brain and reinforce your focus on what you really want: to obtain, maintain, and sustain your desired weight for life.

The exercises are given in hierarchical order. That is, the techniques listed for Week 1 are simpler and more basic than the ones for Week 2, and so on. Each set of techniques builds upon those of the previous week to create a holistic image of your eating patterns. As you become more aware of those patterns, as your left brain becomes more conscious of what you are doing — say, heading for the cookie jar — *when* you are doing it, you will be able to make a conscious choice whether to eat that cookie or wait a while and take a walk first. And as you choose more and more often to take constructive action, your confidence will build and you will discover that you are in control, you are dropping pounds, and the relaxing effects of Reflective Relearning are gradually beginning to replace the old stress-reducing behavior of overeating.

A word of caution: *Give yourself time.* Don't expect instant results or give up when you haven't seen Victoria Principal (or Robert Redford) in the mirror after ten days — or even six weeks, for that matter.

The word "synergy" is helpful in describing how Reflective Relearning works. "Synergy" refers to the idea that the whole is greater than the sum of the parts. As you proceed through the six weeks, remind yourself that the exercises suggested for each week are designed to move you gradually toward a new awareness and appreciation of yourself. Each week builds on the previous one to reinforce your subconscious attention to your eating patterns, which will influence the next week's exercises and strengthen your resolve.

Another thing: *Don't be hard on yourself.* Stop blaming and shaming! Because Reflective Relearning has a cumulative effect, many people become restless after a few days. After the first week or so, the left brain may still be telling you that all of this stuff is a waste of time. After all, it tells you, you have bigger fish to fry (excuse the pun), more important things to do — no time for all of this "consciousness" stuff. Please move past this point. *Fake it till you make it.* After four to six weeks there will be a change, and you will begin to see it manifesting itself in your eating behavior. Even your logical, reasonable left brain will not be able to dismiss the subtle yet undeniable change in your attitude toward eating. Once this attitudinal change sets in, you are on your way to obtaining, maintaining, and sustaining your desired weight forever.

HOW TO FAKE IT TILL YOU MAKE IT

The most difficult part of the Reflective Relearning program is getting the left brain to believe that there is going to be any lasting effect. It is confusing to the left brain to have to wait for the cumulative effect of these exercises to take hold. Many of you might find some of the techniques difficult to "swallow." As for taking it on faith alone, well, your logical side will say "Forget that." You're not alone. Let me share some of the insights that have come from people dealing with the same kind of ambivalence that you might experience.

A gentleman in one of my group sessions declared that he simply could not visualize anything during the "color" exercises (Week 4). He claimed that he saw nothing, that his mind merely wandered aimlessly during the daily ten minutes for the entire week. I showed him some black and white geometric designs and had him stare at them for about a minute. Then I asked him to shut his eyes and see the "negative." This is a natural phenomenon: What was white is now black, and vice versa. He finally got the idea and gradually saw some vague forms. Color, however, was still a problem. One day, during another group session, I suddenly said, "Karl, think of red. What comes to mind?" Without hesitation, he said, "Jaguar." I immediately asked him to shut his eyes and see a red Jaguar. He shut his eyes and literally jumped to his feet, shouting, "Yes, it's there, it's there!" You see, red apples and red flowers meant nothing to him, but a red Jaguar — well, that was a horseless carriage of a different color!

One woman — I'll call her Helen — confided that she simply could not make herself sit still for the daily ten minutes. In session, she asked the group for guidance. Another participant who happened to be a senior citizen shared how she made herself do it: She told herself that she would not get one bite of food until she had done her Reflective Relearning exercise for the entire ten minutes. It had worked for her. The following week, Helen came in, all enthusiastic. She had imposed the same discipline on herself, and, lo and behold, it had worked for her, too. She was pleased and excited, and encouraged everyone else who was having difficulty to do the same. Other new members of the group tried this method for the first few weeks and found that a routine gradually set in, and soon they no longer had to force themselves to sit still for the ten minutes. Reflective Relearning does become easier as it becomes a habit.

Some of my clients have found that the exercises they resist the most involve the mandala or yantra, a symmetrical geometric image on which you will be asked to concentrate in Week 3. Some people's eyes water as if they were crying. Even more difficult than the physical response is the emotional resistance to sitting and focusing on a picture. A solution offered by some members of my groups was that they could "work their way into" this exercise by occasionally shutting their eyes for a few seconds at a time, then returning to the mandala. Gradually, they could go for longer periods without shutting their eyes.

The universal challenge for those who are starting Reflective Relearning is to discipline themselves to select a set time *daily*, in a quiet spot, to do the exercises. Continuity is essential. One woman shared with me that she had done her Reflective Relearn-ing exercises faithfully for the first thirty days and then stopped because of a family crisis. After the crisis passed, she picked up where she had left off and completed her six weeks. The break in the routine, however, left her feeling that she hadn't really mas-tered the Reflective Relearning habit, so she went right back and ran through another six weeks without interruption. This same lady is now wearing a size 9 dress, a size she has not worn since her freshman year in high school. She feels that redoing her entire six-week program without interruption was the turning point, the key to her learning to take control of her eating.

Most of the people with whom I have worked have continued to do some sort of Reflective Relearning exercise daily since com-pleting their initial six-week commitment. They usually take some of the basic ideas of the program and then add their favorite exercise to do over and over. After you do the initial six weeks of exercises in the order outlined here, feel free to use any single technique or a combination of several in the order you choose. If you are anything like the hundreds of overweight people to whom I have taught this method, you will be "hooked" on Reflective Relearning and the beneficial effects it can have, not only on your weight but on many other areas of your life.

For now, remind yourself that you're a beginner. Think of yourself as a budding athlete about to enter six weeks of training. Remind yourself, daily, that this six-week program is *designed* to have a cumulative effect that will be felt gradually. There is no magic pill to whisk you to your goal in a few days, weeks, or even months. Some things in life, usually the most worthwhile ones, take time to achieve — just as it takes approximately nine months for the human fetus to develop into a neonate. So, above all, give yourself time — ten minutes a day, to be precise — to get where you want to be for life.

WEEK 1: TAKE A DEEP BREATH

Each day of this week, you will concentrate on your breathing. The reason I have chosen breathing exercises for this first week is that breathing is the most intimate connection we have with life. Without food, we may live for several weeks. Without water, we could survive for many days. But without air, we may live for only seconds without sustaining brain damage or death.

Breathing has been the subject of much study throughout the ages. The ancients called it *prana*, or life force. As our ancestors experimented with breathing exercises, they discovered many fascinating things. Some experienced spiritual insights, while others found that certain kinds of breathing increased their creativity and lowered their fears and anxieties. Most systems of meditation begin with some sort of breathing exercise. The object of this first week, therefore, is to focus on your breathing and pay attention (consciously) to how your body and thoughts respond at this level of awareness.

On Your Mark

You are in your chosen spot at your designated time of day. (One woman I know likes to do this exercise when she is taking a hot bath. Not only does the warm water help her to relax; she also finds that by sinking her head under the water, she can hear her own breathing better and outside sounds are eliminated.)

Begin by inhaling with "I AM," exhaling with "RELAXED." Do this to the count of three at the start, gradually increasing the number of seconds you sustain each part of the breathing process: "I am (two, three) relaxed (two, three). I am (two, three, four) relaxed (two, three, four)," and so on, until you are able to inhale and exhale to the count of ten. Continue at this level for a minute or so (about three inhale-exhale pairs).

Be sure to say the words "I AM...RELAXED" as you do this exercise. Hear them in your mind if you do not say them aloud. By focusing on these words, you will be quieting your left brain as you move into a more relaxed state. If your left brain does begin to intrude with messages such as "Don't forget to pick up the milk at the store," simply acknowledge the message and then say to yourself, "Now I choose to return to my Reflective Relearning."

This warm-up part of the exercise will take approximately four minutes.

Get Set

After you have completed the warm-up portion and you are breathing deeply and slowly, continue this slow, even breathing as you sink into your relaxed state of awareness. Now allow your muscles to go completely limp. Breathe deeply "into" your muscles, starting with the tips of your toes and moving up to the neck muscles. Feel each muscle "breathing" in time with your own slow breathing.

Next, begin to allow thoughts and images to come to you. Do not try to generate these images. With your eyes closed, view the inside of your eyelids as though they are a television screen. See whatever images or patterns are there. If thoughts accompany these images, fine. Allow them to come and go, but do not try to evaluate them or analyze them. See them nonjudgmentally. In between, continue to listen to your slow, rhythmic breathing. That which we resist will persist, so learn to accept, focus on, and then release the data from the left brain as though you were an outside observer, simply watching your mind at work. Accept whatever comes to you calmly and let it go just as easily.

Another three minutes have passed.

Go!

For the last three minutes, repeat your weight-goal affirmation as outlined in Chapter 7:

"I WILL ALLOW MYSELF TO OBTAIN, MAINTAIN, AND SUSTAIN MY DESIRED WEIGHT OF_____ POUNDS (insert number) BY_____ (insert date and year)."

As you repeat this affirmation to yourself, see the words and numerals written out in bold, capital letters, as though on a large chalkboard or billboard. Repeat the sentence to yourself until you can see this picture clearly.

Reaffirm

Before we end this exercise, I want you to do one more thing:

Say to yourself, "Today, if I have the urge to eat something I really don't want or need, I will sit quietly for one minute and breathe very slowly and very deeply. Then I will repeat my weight goal to myself ten times before I choose whether to eat or not."

This exercise is to be done every day for this first week. When you have completed the exercise, you may wish to record in your journal the images and thoughts that came to you. Do so without trying to assess them — simply keep a record of your inner experiences.

WEEK 2: SOUNDS RIGHT

In this second week, we will focus daily upon a mantra of your choice. A "mantra" is simply a sound, a word, or a series of words that you repeat over and over to yourself. The left brain finds this very dull and boring, rather like driving over flat land for miles and miles with relatively little to look at. The "highway hypnosis" that results is nothing more than the left brain shutting down because it finds the monotony unbearable, which allows the intuitive, creative right side of the brain to become more active, to fill in the gap. It is almost as if the left brain, finding nothing out there to stimulate it, must turn inward to listen to subconscious, right-brain thoughts to keep it going. A mantra works like a monotonous landscape to allow right-brain images to move closer to left-brain, conscious awareness.

It is no surprise, then, that the word "mantra" is related to the Latin word for "mind." Our ancestors were very curious about the mind and studied all its aspects. They found that one way of focusing on it was through invocation or incantation. From a spiritual or religious standpoint, mantras enabled man to focus his mind on the supernatural by inducing a trancelike state and a feeling of connection with otherworldly forces. Many Eastern religions today still use mantras as a means of tuning oneself to the inner mind.

Today, we know from biofeedback that merely repeating the word "relax" over and over to oneself has a great calming effect.

A typical biofeedback machine (which looks like a black box with a dial) indicates states of bodily tension by measuring such things as galvanic skin response. A person hooked up to this machine can become aware of his state of bodily tension and see how it rises and falls with various movements, speech patterns, thoughts, and so on — thereby allowing him to regulate, at least to some extent, his bodily tension. With practice and awareness, he can increase his ability to do this.

In fact, you have already used a type of mantra during your first week of exercises, when you repeated the words "I AM... RELAXED" in time with your slow breathing. Biofeedback has shown that repeating reassuring words to ourselves can enable us to lower our blood pressure, slow down our heart rate, even prevent a migraine headache from occurring. The electronic evidence from biofeedback devices proves this indisputably. How does it work? Who knows? And frankly, for us, who cares? (Your left brain just said, "I care — that's who!"

For our purposes in this second week, we will use a mantra in a rather elementary fashion to disengage the left brain and invoke relaxation of both body and mind. You may choose your own mantra. If you have a strong religious orientation, you may choose a name from your faith, such as Jesus or Buddha, or whatever has special meaning for you. If you do not have this inclination, you may choose any positive word or phrase, such as "happy," "calm," or "I am in control." Or you may wish to try the universal mantra, OM (sounds like "home"), which has been used for centuries. If you use OM, be sure to say it slowly and let the sound resonate through your head cavity. Whatever word or words you decide upon, be sure you are in your private place, where you can say your mantra aloud without people wondering what in the world you are up to.

Stop

Sit quietly in your private place, in a straight-backed chair. Be sure people cannot hear you and disturb you. Breathe quietly and slowly for the first minute while you allow all outside sounds to disappear and you bring the focus inward, with you. All outside sounds should disappear just as they do when you are sleeping, except for loud sounds.

Spend the first three to five minutes saying your mantra aloud, making sure the sounds resonate in your head cavity as long as possible. Say your mantra as long, low, and intensely as you can. Hang on to the last syllable and let it rumble around in your head. Let the sound become part of your being — not just your head but your entire being. Of course, the left brain will turn on from time to time just to let you know how crazy it thinks this entire thing is. Accept its input and again consciously *will* your awareness into the mantra. You have completed this step when the mantra is all there is and you are physically and mentally united with it.

Look

When you are completely one with your mantra, begin to focus on your bodily sensations as you continue saying your mantra. Is there some tension? Are your legs cramped? Is your stomach growling? What are the somatic (physical) signs? Once you note them, release them immediately. Say to yourself, "Yes, my stomach is growling — I'll tend to that later. Now I consciously choose to direct my will back into my mantra."

After rejoining your mantra for another minute or so, begin to allow food thoughts and images to come to you. Again, put them on your mental "TV monitor" and simply let them be. Allow the sounds and various meanings of your mantra to call up whatever images and attitudes about food and eating come to you. See them and appreciate them, but do not judge them. For example, if you are using the word "joy" as your mantra, you may begin to see images of an ice cream sundae or a black, slinky, size 6 dress. It doesn't matter — simply notice the images on the screen of your subconsciousness, then release them as they suggest new thoughts and images, and watch those.

When no images or thoughts appear, go back to focusing on your mantra and listening to it, merging with it. *Never attempt to force yourself to have thoughts or see images.* If you do, you are using your left brain and shutting out all of those interesting things your right brain and subconscious mind hold for you. Believe me, by the end of the week your right-brain thoughts and images will be surfacing independently of your left brain. They will seem to come to you unbidden, as though they emanated from somewhere outside. If this doesn't happen right away, do not try to make it happen. Simply continue saying your mantra. This step has taken about four minutes.

And Listen

Finally, spend the last three to five minutes repeating your weight-goal affirmation:

"I WILL ALLOW MYSELF TO OBTAIN, MAINTAIN, AND SUSTAIN MY DESIRED WEIGHT OF _____ POUNDS BY _____ ."

If, during any day in this second week, you have the urge to eat something you do not want or need, sit for one minute in your private place and repeat your mantra to yourself, focusing during alternate repetitions of your mantra on the food you want to eat and then on your weight goal. You are now ready to make a clearheaded decision about whether to eat the food.

Repeat this exercise every day during this second week of Reflective Relearning. As the week progresses, you will find that the initial phase of the exercise, becoming "one" with your mantra, is easier and takes place sooner. You will also find that subconscious thoughts and right-brain images of food and eating will come to the surface more quickly and more intensely, and that different images will follow, one upon the other, with greater rapidity. Again, "go with the flow." Do not attempt to judge. Do, however, record your experience in your journal.

WEEK 3: PICTURE THIS

This week we are going to concentrate on a mandala, or, as some call it, a "yantra." The mandala or yantra is a symmetrical geometric picture designed to frustrate the left brain. The left brain finds spatial relationships difficult to deal with and thus eventually becomes bored and stops paying attention. This frees your right-brain images and subconscious thoughts to come to the surface.

Like the mantra, the mandala or yantra is an ancient concept. Early man recognized his need for creative expression as well as for symmetry and wholeness. The mandala fulfilled this need with its pleasing, balanced symmetry that contained intricate, complex patterns. This complex yet uniform image offered a sort of comfort. Perhaps it even met some basic need in early man for a sense of control over his universe and a feeling of balance in his life. Modern experience confirms this impression: When we take a few moments out of our day to contemplate some visually perfect object (such as a candle or a flower), there is a marked calming effect on the body that may be measured as reduced blood pressure or slower breathing.

Some examples of simple mandalas are presented in the next few pages. You can use any of them for the exercises this week, or you may wish to create and color your own, a rewarding experience in itself. If you like, you may choose to use several different mandalas — the results are much the same. You may find, however, that some are more pleasing to your eye and easier to concentrate on than others.

You may be surprised to discover that this week's lesson in visual focusing is more tasking than the lessons of the first two weeks. During the first week, you were asked only to attend to your breathing. Week 2 was slightly more complex, as you concentrated upon a specific audio stimulation. The visual pattern on which you focus this week will take more stamina and will call up more complex (and interesting) mental responses, but after two weeks of flexing your right-brain muscles your mind should be ready to exert itself a bit. After all, you're in training!

Star of Wonder

Sit comfortably in a chair and hold the mandala of your choice. You don't need to think about what you are doing; just keep your eyes focused on the center of the design and "sense" what is

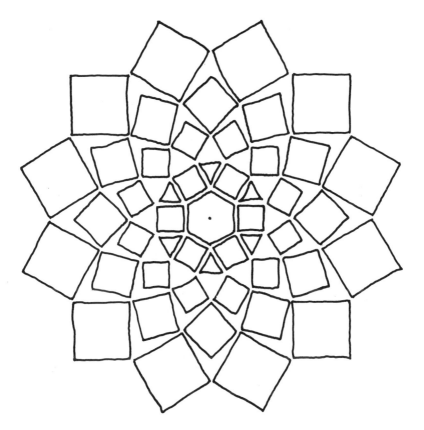

Mandala 1

happening. Look at the center of the design as long as you feel comfortable doing so. If your eyes begin to water or you become fatigued, simply close your eyes and rest them for a few moments; then return to the process. Do this for at least three minutes at the beginning, working up to five minutes by the end of the week.

During the second and remaining days of the week, the mandala should begin to call forth subconscious thoughts and right-brain images. Become increasingly aware of how the forms seem to change. Deliberately focus on the center for a minute. Then

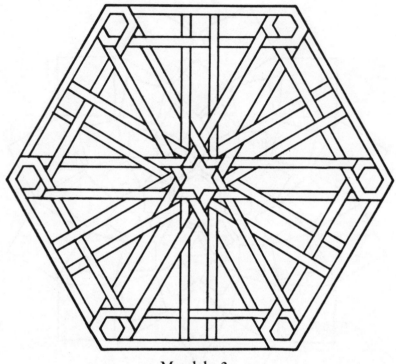

Mandala 2

shift your focus to the black spaces for another minute. Finally, focus on the white. As you do so, you will notice that the mandala seems to move, the pattern swimming or spinning around the center or the white or black spaces "popping up" and radiating outward to fill your visual screen and blur into shifting forms. When you need to rest your eyes, you will find that, upon closing them, a negative of the mandala appears on the insides of your eyelids.

As the minutes go by, you should begin to become "one" with your mandala, just as you became one with your mantra. Whatever thoughts come to you, simply say to yourself, "Yes, that thought is there," and then make a conscious decision to release the thought and return to concentrating on the mandala. Imagine that you are falling toward the center of the mandala, as though it were a long tunnel with the center at its end. Allow the mandala to envelop you. Be it, feel it, flow with it. You have become one with your mandala when you are "standing" at its center and its patterns are surrounding you, swirling about you.

Star of Light

Still focusing on the mandala, begin to tune in to your bodily sensations. Moving from toes to head, consciously release all tension you find in each portion of your body: Uncurl your toes; allow your calves and thighs to go limp; feel your back muscles loosen from the base of your spine upward to your shoulder and neck muscles; let the tightness drain from jaws, eyes, and forehead. Do this for one minute.

Now, for another minute or two, continue to focus on your mandala as you allow its shapes to suggest images of your body as you expect it to be. Again, do not force yourself (that is, do not use your left brain) to come up with images. Simply hold the concept of "body" in mind as you stare at your mandala and allow it to suggest shapes corresponding to your own human form as it can be. You may, for example, see yourself looking great in that sexy bathing suit from last week's spring sportswear catalog. Whatever you "see," my only requirement is that you focus on what *makes you feel good.*

I'm the Star I See Tonight

The last phase of this week's exercise is, again, your weight-goal affirmation:

"I WILL ALLOW MYSELF TO OBTAIN, MAINTAIN, AND SUSTAIN MY DESIRED WEIGHT OF _____ POUNDS BY _____ ."

Continue to concentrate on your mandala as you say your affirmation to yourself, seeing any images that relate to your desired bodily form.

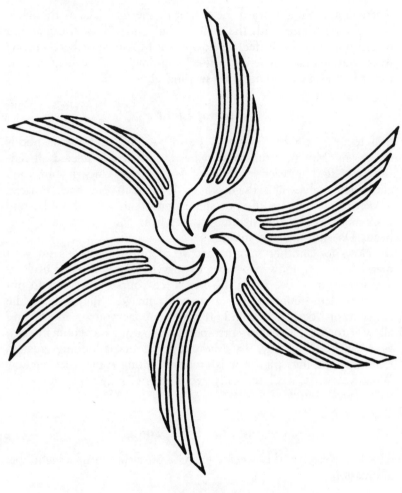

Mandala 3

This week, when you find yourself heading for the refrigerator when you're not really hungry, grab your mandala and focus on it for one minute. Then choose.

As you repeat your exercise with the mandala, you will find your concentration growing and your eyestrain diminishing. By the end of the week, merging with the mandala will have become much easier and quicker, and the bodily images it suggests in your right brain will surface with increasing rapidity. Again, allow these images to come and go as quickly as they will, and constantly focus on the mandala — even during your weight-goal affirmation.

WEEK 4: OVER THE RAINBOW

Well, you are halfway finished with your six-week training program. Are you proud of yourself for "hanging in there"? You should be. The hardest part is over. If you've faithfully stuck it out for twenty-one consecutive days, you are beginning to notice the beneficial effects of Reflective Relearning, not only on your nerves but also on your food-related thinking patterns. You are now highly aware of each misdirected step you take toward the kitchen, and by now you are deciding, not just sliding, when it comes to whether (or what) to eat. The next three weeks will be a piece of cake. (Who said that?!)

In the fourth week, we move up the hierarchical scale to a slightly more complex series of exercises. This week we will be examining color. The ancients had some very strange and wonderful ideas about colors and their connection with specific energy centers of the body, or "chakras." Some of our medicine-men ancestors claimed to be able to "read auras," or "see" the various colors emanating from different parts of the body. They interpreted these auras as revealing various states of energy and health. In modern times, the calming effects of focusing on certain colors in connection with certain parts of the body have been scientifically documented. Certain individuals are able to execute amazing feats (such as slowing their heart rates significantly) while focusing on specific colors and chakras.

The exercises for this week have been broken down by day. Each day we will focus on a different color associated with a different energy level or state of awareness. At the end of each exercise, as you have every day during the course of this program, spend the last three to five minutes repeating your weight-goal affirmation:

"I WILL ALLOW MYSELF TO OBTAIN, MAINTAIN, AND SUSTAIN MY DESIRED WEIGHT OF _____ POUNDS BY _____ ."

Day 1

Today, I want you to think of the color red. Red is associated with the most primary emotions — reminiscent of blood, fire, the physical, the animal, and the primordial. Feel this red centered about the base of your spine. Think "into" the red and let it fill the base of your spine for three to five minutes. As you continue to hold on to the red and center it about the base of your spine, red objects may come to you: an apple, a flower, even a red Jaguar. Melt these objects into the base of your spine and hold the red there. As always, acknowledge and quickly release any left-brain thoughts that intrude.

At the end of this first phase, hold the red while you repeat your weight-goal affirmation for the remaining five minutes of your session.

Day 2

Our color today is orange, a color that moves us from the physical to a transitional realm between the physical and the emotional. Let orange come into your awareness. Once you "lock" this color in your mind, let it center itself about your navel region, encircling the entire lower abdomen. Please don't worry if you don't actually see the color orange. Just hold the thought — eventually the color will come. After three to five minutes of holding the orange about your lower abdomen, you are ready to return to your final five minutes of weight-goal affirmation. Retain the orange and see your affirmation written in that color.

Day 3

Today our color is yellow. Like orange, this color is at the "gut level" — transitional, yet more associated with the emotions than with the physical. Allow yellow objects to come to your mind:

yellow daisies, the sun, a yellow shirt, and so on. Now let that yellow center itself in your diaphragm — right in the solar plexus, right in the center of your being. Hold this yellow at your center for three to five minutes before going on to your affirmation for the remaining five minutes. Play around with the numbers you have set for your weight goal and see if you can get them to come to you in yellow.

Day 4

Now we move to green and to a higher center of the body, the heart. The association of both the heart and the color green with life and growth is an ancient one. Likewise, we are right at the center of the emotions here — halfway between the purely physical and the purely intellectual.

Think of green grass, green money, "green" youth. Once you have thought of all the green objects or ideas you can, melt this color into a single green and center it about your heart area. Feel its richness sinking into and emanating out from your heart in time with your heartbeat. Sink your entire being into your heart and the green that envelops it. Be green. Merge with green. When you have "become" green, spend the final five minutes of the session repeating your affirmation to yourself — in green, if it will come that way.

Day 5

Today we are going to focus on blue — a very cool, calming color, which we will center on the throat and neck, the site of a great deal of tension for many people (especially those who pass too much food through it). Again, begin by thinking of everything you can that is blue: blue skies, blue wildflowers, blue water. When you are swimming in blue, focus it into your neck. Feel blue emanating from your throat and speech area. Let it cool your neck and throat for five minutes. The whole world is blue — just blue. Stay in blue as you complete the initial five minutes and move into your five-minute affirmation.

Day 6

Today we are going to concentrate on purple, a very regal color. Think of a king's purple velvet robe, purple lilacs, purple grapes. Now focus that purple on your "third eye" — that spot right between and above your eyebrows, in the middle of your forehead. Many cultures believe that this spot is the "eye of God," the focal point of spirituality in man, and that concentrating on this area can heighten awareness and bring about change. Let purple encircle your "third eye"; feel it emanating from the middle of your forehead and merge with it, sinking deeply into it. The self-confidence and regalness of this color should accompany you into your last five minutes of weight-goal affirmation.

Day 7

For this final day, we will focus on a color that is really not a color at all but, appropriately, a merging of all colors: white. White is representative of the higher mind — an accumulation of all that is physical, emotional, intellectual, and spiritual. It is very bright, very alive, associated with clarity and light.

See white lights — incandescent, fluorescent, stagelights, headlights, street lights, candlelight, moonlight, starlight. Allow the white light to begin to revolve around your body, as though you were the sun giving out all this brightness. The white emanates from your head and mind, lighting up everything around you and eventually becoming so bright that everything is overcome by this blinding light. Stay in this vast lightness for one or two minutes. Then allow your affirmation to begin as you bask in white. Spend the next five minutes successfully reprogramming yourself to obtain, maintain, and sustain your desired weight for life.

During this week, when you feel the urge to eat, stop first to focus on the color of the day and its related chakra. Concentrate this color into its seat in the body for one minute before making your *choice* of whether to eat.

WEEK 5: THANKS FOR THE MEMORY

For your exercises this week, you will draw upon images and thoughts that are both more complex and more familiar than those of the previous weeks. These exercises are fun and also will probably bring back some long-forgotten memories. Remember the television show *This Is Your Life*? Well, this is sorta like that. I will ask you to trace certain times in your life. Some of these may be unpleasant. If you find that a memory on which you are focusing is uncomfortable, please turn to another, more pleasant time in your life. The purpose here is to draw on positive memories, not painful ones.

On the scale of difficulty, Week 5 is tougher than anything you've experienced yet. Your first four weeks, however, have made this process possible. Current research confirms that when people are more relaxed, calmer, and more in control, their recall of earlier events is much greater. It is difficult to recall past events when current events in our lives are making us anxious or nervous. High-level anxiety blocks memory — ask any student who is about to take a BIG test. When anxiety levels drop, recall is greater and much more vivid. Now that you have learned to tune in to deeper levels of awareness of yourself, you are going to find that some of your "mental blocks" to memory have faded and your capacity for recall is greater than it was when you began this program.

Again, as in Week 4, the exercises are broken down by day. Each day, you will be asked to focus upon a specific memory. The seven exercises are designed to help you gain new insights into your personality development and its relationship to your current eating behavior.

Day 1

As usual, we begin by quieting the left brain and enhancing the ease with which your right-brain images and subconscious thoughts come to the surface. For the first minute or so, sit quietly in a straight-backed chair and breathe very deeply. Let the air pass through your nostrils gently and fully. Inhale deeply, all the way down to your stomach, making sure the lungs are as full as possible. Then exhale slowly, emptying every last bit of carbon dioxide.

Now, I want you to reflect a long way back. Find the first memory you have of being alive, the earliest memory you can recall. Find it without too much searching — don't allow the left brain to say, "Well, maybe there's something in there that's even earlier." Simply focus on the earliest memory that comes to mind. Where were you? How old were you? Who was with you? What were you wearing? Hold this memory for at least three minutes, allowing as much detail to surface as you can. Let it be there. Reflect upon it. Accept new dimensions of it.

At the end of this phase slowly release the memory, as you use the next five minutes to repeat your weight-goal affirmation. Pay close attention to your visual image of the affirmation written before you. It is probably much clearer than it was a few weeks ago. If the numerals representing your desired weight and the date by which you wish to obtain that weight are fairly clear now, then concentrate on seeing your body at that weight — the way it will soon look.

Day 2

Again, begin by sitting quietly and breathing deeply to attain a relaxed state. Make your mind as blank as possible. Look at your mental "TV screen," but don't turn it on. Imagine you are looking at the blank screen.

Now return to your childhood. Remember your favorite toy. Please take the first toy that pops into your mind, even if your logical left brain might object that it wasn't necessarily your favorite toy. If you have trouble recalling a toy, recall a favorite pet. Just take the toy or pet that comes to you — remember, your right brain stores special events from childhood just as your left brain does. When did you get this toy or pet? Who gave it to you? Did others play with it along with you? How did it make you feel? When the object or animal becomes fully realized in your mind, allow it to remain there for three or four minutes.

As you release the image of your favorite toy or pet and enter your five minutes of weight-goal affirmation, concentrate on seeing your body in a particular outfit that you would like to wear.

Day 3

Today, we are going to go back into your childhood to recall the very first friend you ever had. Sit quietly for the first minute to "breathe" yourself into a relaxed state as you let this friend come to mind. Who was this friend? Male or female? Was the friend a neighbor? Were your parents friends with the child's parents? Where did you live at the time? Where did your friend live? Hold these memories for the next three or four minutes. Don't strain — let them come to you and grow at their own pace.

Now, take the next five minutes for the important task of reprogramming yourself to obtain, maintain, and sustain your desired weight for life. Again, if the numerals which represent your desired weight are clear, focus on seeing your body as you desire it to be. Imagine that you are with a current good friend, sharing how good it feels to be at your desired weight.

Day 4

Sit comfortably for one minute with your mind as blank as you can make it and your breathing rhythmic and full. Go back in your memory and recall the first day you went to school. It may be preschool, kindergarten, or first grade — take any day that *first* comes to you. It is important to let this first memory come in and to allow your visual recall to elaborate on it without judgment from your conscious mind and left brain. Recall the teacher. Male or female? Pretty/handsome? Can you see any of the other children with you? Do you remember your first reading book? Recess games? An art project? Hold this memory for at least four minutes, allowing flashes of these early school memories to come and go.

As you release your school memories, entering your affirmation phase, visualize yourself at your desired weight, doing an activity you would like to do with some of your friends. Dress yourself appropriately for this occasion, whether it be in a swimsuit for the beach or an evening outfit for a concert.

Day 5

Take your first minute to move into your relaxed, right-brain state. Breathe deeply; set aside worries and concerns.

Now allow a group of people to form in your mind. You are a child again, and you are at a family gathering. The mood is festive — relatives and friends are gathered together to celebrate a special event. What is the occasion? Christmas? A wedding reception? A graduation? Where are you? In your parents home? At a church? At school? Who is there? List as many of the people as you can recall. Were there other children? Cousins? A best friend? Did you play with these other children?

There is food — a meal or a buffet prepared especially for this occasion. What are some of the foods? What are your favorites? What did you eat? Where did you eat — with grown-ups, or separately, with the other children? How much did you eat? How did you feel after eating? Just right? Too full?

Now move from these memories to your weight-goal affirmation, repeating your goal to yourself for the final five minutes of the session. As you do so, think of how you feel after eating a meal — either with others or alone. How does this feeling compare with the way you felt after eating at that special gathering years ago?

Day 6

Once again, clear your mind by breathing deeply for a minute. Let no worries or thoughts intrude — you're going to have fun, and I want you to be ready for it. Think back to a very special day in your past — this time, a day that was devoted to a special activity or outing. Take the *first* day that comes to you. Got it? Okay, that's it — no more scanning with your left brain for special days. If you came up with an immediate visual impression of a special day, that means your right brain thought it was pretty special. What was the activity? A trip to the beach? To an amusement park? To a concert? What were you wearing? Who was with you? What did you do? Allow the details to accumulate as you enjoy this for three or four minutes.

Release the memory as you enter your affirmation phase. This time, as you see yourself at your desired weight, fantasize, in detail, that you are engaging in a special activity with a special friend. What are you wearing? Where are you? Is it summer, winter? Evening, morning?

Day 7

Today is your last trip down memory lane for this week. Take a minute to move into your relaxed, self-aware state. (It's becoming easier and easier, isn't it?) Now, quietly reflect on a *recent* happy occasion, preferably within the last few months. Again, take the first thing that comes, trusting your right-brain, visual storehouse to know when you were happy. How did you feel? Who was with you? What were you doing that caused your pleasure? Let it all come easily and slowly — no need to force it. Re-create the pleasurable occasion as you hold these thoughts for three or four minutes.

This time, as you make your weight-goal affirmation, I want you to imagine a similar happy occasion that you might bring about with the new confidence and self-love instilled by your newfound self-control and your increasingly pleasing body form. Make a plan. What will the occasion be? A party you plan to throw? A night at the theater? A trip to that art festival next weekend? Who will be with you? How will you feel? What are some of the things you can do to bring this occasion about?

WEEK 6: A LITTLE HELP FROM MY FRIENDS

Well, here we are in the final week of training. If you've made it this far (and I always knew you would), be proud of you. Your attitudes about eating have begun to change, slowly but surely. Notice how much calmer you are than you were five weeks ago, not to mention how much better you are at concentrating on all sorts of things, not just your exercises.

Speaking of exercises, let's do a few more before I let you fly to continue on your own. This week, you will incorporate some visual, auditory, imaginative techniques to obtain not only your desired weight but also some answers for yourself. Predictably, this series of exercises is the most complex and sophisticated of the lot, but also the most fun and childlike. The next seven days offer a real playground for your mind. When we were children, we played constantly and easily. As adults, playing often becomes hard "work," since we allow fears of being foolish or preoccupations with the daily challenges of job and family to interfere with our natural gift for play. That's the left brain again: You don't have time for such wasteful foolishness, it says. Some left brains never know when to take a vacation!

At this point, you have taught your left brain a little about how to relax, so the next week of exercises shouldn't come as a great shock to it. Instead, these seven lessons may well be the most enjoyable and powerful ones you've experienced yet. That's why they're placed here in the sixth week — a sort of dessert. (Oops!)

As always, it is very important for you to accept what comes to you — perhaps more important now than in any of the earlier weeks. Judgments and evaluations must be suspended. You've had five weeks to learn to do this, so don't be surprised if you get some pretty heavy-duty insights. Listen to what your right brain reveals to you as though you were a bystander, interested but not involved in its messages. Unless you have had classes in guided imagery, have been in psychotherapy or engaged in some other self-revelatory process, you might find that many of them have not surfaced before. This week will assist you in focusing on your innermost desires and discovering what it takes for you to be *fulfilled*, not filled full. Learn from these experiences as you take greater and greater control over your eating patterns. You are in charge now.

Day 1

Clear your mind as you go into your first minute of deep relaxation. You are a pro at this now, so I won't remind you again that it is the first step of each daily session. I'll assume that you're into your right-brain state, breathing deeply and ready to accept what comes.

Now, I want you to let your imagination take over completely. Imagine a room made just for you. Design your own furniture. Decorate this place to your exact taste. Make it any size you wish, and put as many objects in the room as you like. Let yourself go wild with colors, fabrics, materials, artwork, flowers, sculpture, high-tech equipment — whatever you like. Work on your room for three or four minutes, and then take an extra minute to stand back and admire your artistic handiwork. See yourself sitting in *your* room in *your* favorite chair, completely relaxed and in control of your life.

As you relax in that favorite chair, begin your five minutes of saying to yourself:

"I WILL ALLOW MYSELF TO OBTAIN, MAINTAIN, AND SUSTAIN MY DESIRED WEIGHT OF _____ POUNDS BY _____ ."

Think of how much your body form will please you as you sit in your perfect room.

Day 2

Today, re-create your perfect room and hold the image in your mind for thirty seconds or so. Now, imagine the doorbell ringing and a very special person entering the room as you answer the door. This person is very wise and knows every desire you have — even some that you are unaware of at this time. See this person clearly. Is he or she someone you know or someone you have never seen before? How is this person dressed? Look at the face closely. Know that this person knows something about you that you probably don't understand at this time. Just let the person be there with you in your special room for the remaining three or four minutes. Hold the picture in your mind as clearly as possible as you return to your weight-goal affirmation, and visualize yourself looking exactly the way you wish to look.

Day 3

Re-create your special room and your wise person. Today, I want you to approach this wise person and ask him or her if you may seek some important answers regarding your life. Wait to see if this person agrees. If so, begin by asking this person to reveal to you what you need to understand about your weight. Ask this question:

"WHAT IS THE MEANING OF MY CURRENT WEIGHT?"

Let the answers come to you without any judgment or any type of censorship. Just be there and receive the answers. Your wise person is responding without criticism — in a loving, caring way. Let this happen. Let go and hear what this wise person has to say. Hold these answers in your mind as you complete your session with your affirmation that you will obtain, maintain, and sustain your desired weight.

Day 4

Again, quickly re-create your special room and your wise person. First, thank this person for the time he or she spent with you yesterday. Let your wise person know that you appreciate the advice and accept it without judgment or stipulations. Let this person know that you completely trust him or her to guide you to the answers that lie deep within you. These insights may have been withheld from your conscious mind and left brain because of fear, doubt, self-hate, whatever. You are now thanking this person for releasing these insights into your consciousness.

Today, ask this special person what emotions you need to release from your life. Ask this question:

"AM I HOLDING ANY RESENTMENT, ANGER, FRUS-
TRATION, OR OTHER FEELING THAT HAMPERS MY
TOTAL WELL-BEING?"

Listen to what the wise person has to say. Let go of any of the

negative emotions he or she tells you to release. Think of someone you resent. Let that person go. Think of someone who has
hurt you in the past. Let him or her go. Hanging on to these
negative emotions drains your precious energy. You now need
this energy to gain your desired weight and live a productive,
fulfilling life. Thank your special person and tell him or her that
you'll get back together tomorrow. Enter your weight-affirmation
phase as you release negative emotions, and continue for five
minutes to the end of your session.

Day 5

You are back in your special room with your special person.
Again, thank that person for yesterday's help, knowing that the
insights you have gained contain no criticism or condemnation.
Recall these insights as you ask your special person a new
question:

"WHAT DO I NEED TO DO IN ORDER TO BE MORE
CREATIVE?"

Let the person talk freely now. Don't interrupt. Listen to everything this person says without labeling it as crazy, too hard, "not
like me," too expensive, or stupid. Just *listen.* Listen and grow.
Listen and gain valuable insights into your creativity. If the person
suggests that you paint or write or join a baseball team, just soak
it up.

Hold some of your wise person's suggestions in mind as you
enter and complete your self-affirmation. See yourself enacting
some of these suggestions at your desired weight.

Day 6

You are back in your special room, with your special person, and
you are expressing your appreciation for yesterday's insights. Today
you are going to ask this person a very important question. It is
imperative that you receive the answers nonjudgmentally and
without resistance. Ask the following question:

"WHAT IS IT THAT I NEED TO BE _FULFILLED_ IN MY LIFE?"

Now be quiet and listen. Let the answers come freely and at their own pace. Do not try to make them up yourself. Listen and wait for the answers as you look intently into this person's face, see the facial expressions, and observe the body gestures. As the answers come, absorb them, repeating them after your wise person in your own tone of voice. Thank this person for these insights.

Now spend the final five minutes of your session repeating to yourself:

"I WILL ALLOW MYSELF TO OBTAIN, MAINTAIN, AND SUSTAIN MY DESIRED WEIGHT OF _____ POUNDS BY _____ ."

Day 7

This is the last "official" day of your exercises. Most people by now feel much more familiar with the process. Naturally, your left-brain, verbal side still interrupts from time to time, but you have learned how to handle it quickly and effectively. You have also become an expert at moving yourself into a state of complete relaxation.

On this last day of training, go back to your special room with your wise person. Thank that person for the valuable insights imparted yesterday, and ask if you may make one more request. If the person agrees, ask the following questions:

"WHAT ELSE DO I NEED TO KNOW ABOUT MY WEIGHT? IS THERE SOMETHING I NEED TO KNOW SO AS TO MOVE QUICKLY TOWARD MY DESIRED WEIGHT?"

Now, sit quietly and again do not force an answer to come. Something will come. Listen until it does; do not induce it yourself. Simply let the process unfold. When the answer does come, do not judge it. Say nothing, either to your wise person or to yourself. Simply thank that person (don't say goodbye) and move on to your Reflective Relearning affirmation.

KEEPING THE FAITH

It is fascinating to me that, as I was about to begin writing this chapter, I received a call from a lady — I'll call her Denise — who had taken a class from me. She told me that she had purchased my tapes on weight control, *Leaving Your Fat Behind,* and had used them faithfully for about six days. Then "something" came up, and she skipped a day. Next, she skipped two, and finally she fell off the proverbial wagon. Sound familiar? It does to me, too — I've been there. It is so easy to slip into negative patterns, especially when the left-brain, "sane" side of us urges us not to waste time on such craziness as Reflective Relearning.

At any rate, Denise had called to tell me that she had stopped doing these exercises and had stopped listening to the tapes — and in general had gone back to "business as usual." Then, six months later, one of her sons came home from college with a friend of his and was excitedly telling this friend how his mother controlled her weight through Reflective Relearning. Denise was embarrassed, as it was obvious that she wasn't controlling anything about her weight.

After her son returned to college, Denise got back to business and faithfully did her exercises for ten minutes daily. She also did her power-walking (see Chapter 10) for thirty to forty minutes a day. She had called me to say that after that day in June, when her son reminded her of the Reflective Relearning process, she could proudly say that she had moved twenty-three pounds nearer to her desired weight. She said she just wanted me to know that she was only six pounds away from her goal weight and hadn't a doubt that she would be there soon. She also laughingly told me that her son and his friend were once again home for the holidays, and her son had remarked that, obviously, his "reverse psychology" was working for her! One thing Denise also told me was that, although she had done her Reflective Relearning process for only a few days six months before, she felt there was a cumulative effect because she got back into the exercises very quickly and with firm determination.

One man who was particularly resistant to giving ten minutes of his busy schedule to Reflective Relearning serves as an excellent example of how hanging in there pays off. He was sent to me by his cardiologist because of an irregular EKG and his excessive poundage. The first thing he told me was that he didn't really care about his weight as far as his looks were concerned. At the age of 52, being forty-six pounds overweight did not bother him. I asked if he wanted to live to be 53. He was aghast. Of course he did, he said. I looked him straight in the eye and said, "Well, prove it." From that point on, he was determined to show me how faithful he could be to this "stupid" program. He was truly angry and resistant in the first place, and it was delightful to see these emotions melt into sheer amazement and almost reverence. After four weeks, he had referred three of his buddies to me and was interested in using the Reflective Relearning process to lower his blood pressure. He successfully reduced his weight and blood pressure, and his EKG became much more normal. Today, he is an ardent fan of Reflective Relearning — there's no better spokesman than a convert! He's still doing his ten or twenty minutes daily, he feels wonderful, and says he's shooting for 103, not just 53!

So can you. No one knows better than I do how difficult it can be to convince the logical, critical left brain of the importance and effectiveness of allowing our right-brain knowingness to manifest itself and work for us in our daily lives. As I say, I've been there, and I've seen many others — many of them facing situations that are more life-threatening than obesity — who have been there, too. So let me close out this chapter with just one more story from my files.

A few years back, I worked with a lady who had been actively suicidal and had undergone a great many hospitalizations for attempted suicide. She came to me with very little hope. I asked that she dedicate six weeks to working with me and that she do the Reflective Relearning exercises faithfully for that period of time. She agreed, and we began working together. She saw me twice a week for the next six weeks. Each week, I asked if she was doing her exercises, each week she said "yes," and each week she insisted that nothing had changed. Week after week, the same story. She swore that NOTHING had changed and that she was still depressed and contemplating suicide.

Finally, in the sixth week, I confronted her. I asked her to think of *anything* that might be an indication that she was less depressed and less concerned with suicide. She thought for a minute, and then looked at me with amazement. She said that she had just then realized (comes the dawn!) that for the first time on her way to the session she hadn't considered driving her car off the road and over a cliff (she had to come over some rather winding, high roads to get to my office). I asked her what she felt about that, and she simply shrugged her shoulders.

I had to work with her for several more sessions to convince her that this was a gigantic step forward. She had become so accustomed to feeling suicidal that when the obsession stopped for one day, she almost dismissed this progress as "coincidental." It is amazing how the verbal left brain will take over and rationalize thoughts and behavior that emanate from the right brain. This woman turned out to be more motivated than she thought possible, and once she saw that the process of Reflective Relearning was really working, she really took to the program whole-heartedly. She not only stopped ruminating about suicide but even got a part-time job in a woman's clothing store and loved it. She now sends me a Christmas card every year, in which she sings the praises of her daily reflective exercises. She says that she will never stop doing those exercises, which, in her case, were literally a lifesaver.

In your case, I hope the threat to life is not so obvious. Yet I have worked with many, many people who have overcome obsessional eating through Reflective Relearning and have told me that the process indeed saved their lives, not only emotionally but physically as well. It is very exciting to see people actually changing their lives right before your eyes. I am sure you can do it, too.

As you have moved through the six-week program outlined in this chapter, you have heard the conscious, "smart" side of you telling you to come to your senses and give up all this airy-fairy stuff. You may still be getting some of these messages as you continue the Reflective Relearning process on your own. But one thing's for sure: You now know that the "reasonable" part of you, the part that tells you to give up, is just that — only a part of you. You also know that there is another side which has induced the attitudinal changes you've experienced over the past six weeks. It is telling you to forge ahead to smaller and better things. Keep listening to it every day, for at least ten minutes. It holds the secrets that will allow you to obtain, maintain, and sustain your desired weight for life.

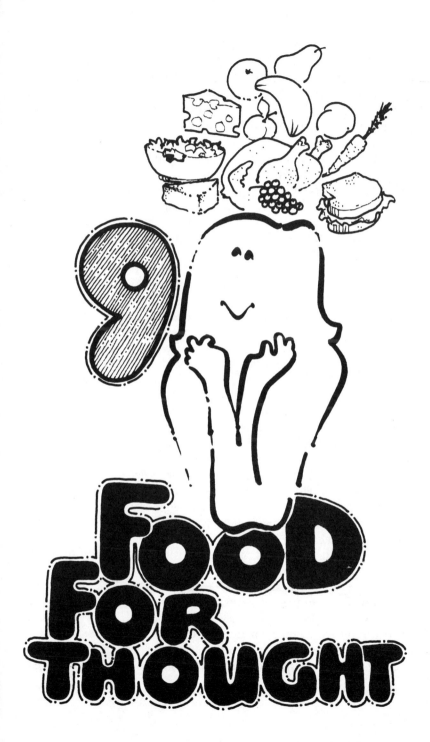

9

FOOD FOR THOUGHT

WE HAVE BEEN CONCENTRATING THROUGHOUT THIS BOOK on how to bring our right-brain, subconscious drives to consciousness so that we can choose patterns of behavior that will help us to obtain, maintain, and sustain our desired weight.

Now that you have faithfully followed your "introductory" six-week program of Reflective Relearning (and you are still doing your ten minutes a day, right?), you have become more expert at recognizing, consciously, why you eat. This new awareness, in turn, has allowed you to make conscious decisions about your eating behavior. Rather than letting your subconscious "automatic pilot" direct your hand toward the cookie jar without "you" thinking about it, you (and your left brain) are now more connected with "yourself" (and your right brain), to the point where you (all of you) are in control, and you are making the choices.

No more digging into the ice cream carton when the kids are impossible. Now you are choosing courses of action that not only help you to meet your weight challenge but also help you to resolve the emotional challenges that used to prompt overeating. To the cue: "I'm angry (or bored or whatever)," you now respond, "so what do I need to do to deal with my anger?" You may *choose* to take a walk to "cool off," or make a plan to confront Billy about his homework, or go to the yarn shop to pick out those beautiful mauve hues for that afghan you've been wanting to crochet for your bedroom. Rather than ignoring your needs by "filling full" (and causing yourself more grief in the long run), you are now fulfilling your needs — directly, consciously, by *choice*. The dual benefit is that you are simultaneously moving closer to your desired weight. This "killing two birds with one stone" process is the beauty of Reflective Relearning.

Yet it's still tough — I know — to deal with food. After all, you may not live to eat anymore, but you still need to eat to live. Making the transition from food-as-comforter to food-as-nourishment can be a source of confusion and anxiety for those of us who have used food as the answer to emotional needs. Let's face it: You can't stop eating for the rest of your life. The big question is: How do you eat appropriately, to fuel yourself for all those exciting activities (and, yes, confrontations with daily challenges) that fulfill your needs and your life? In this chapter we're going to engage in a bit of straight "food talk": Where have you been? Where are you going? and What strategies can you use to develop new eating behaviors? With a little conscious effort on the part of your left brain and patient application over time you can transform these strategies into right-brain, subconscious habits that will allow you to obtain, maintain, and sustain your desired weight.

WHERE WE'VE BEEN: THE HAZARDS OF THE AFFLUENT DIET

As you read in Chapter 4, being fat or thin is partly a matter of culture. Today, most people in Western industrialized nations eat an "affluent" diet consisting of large amounts of animal proteins and fats (meat and dairy products), highly refined flours and sugars (instead of the bulky carbohydrates found in whole grains, tubers, fresh fruits and vegetables), and commercially processed "fast" foods (instead of fresh, unprocessed foods). Such a diet is low in fiber and high in fat. In fact, about 50% of the calories in a North American's diet are fats, as compared to less than 25% for those living in poorer countries. Much of this fat comes from our high consumption of red meat (beef and pork rather than poultry and fish): Americans consume close to 250 POUNDS of red meat per person per year. In poorer countries, that figure can be less than 20 pounds.

When combined with our predominantly sedentary lifestyles, this diet leads to obesity, which encourages diabetes, hypertension, coronary artery disease, diverticulosis, and cancer of the bowel, breast, and prostrate. In a culture that eats so high on the food chain, it's no wonder that many of us are fat — and risking our lives. Consider these facts:

— High consumption of cholesterol-rich foods can raise cholesterol levels in the blood by 10%. Of the coronary deaths in North America and Europe, 10% are people under the age of 55; over 50% of coronary deaths are people under age 75.

— In the United States, between 10% and 20% of children are overweight; the figure ranges from 35% to 50% for middle-aged people.

— In New York City, a study found that one-third of lower-class women are overweight, and one-twentieth of upper-class women are overweight.

— Men who are 10% overweight have a one-third greater chance of dying prematurely from ailments such as heart disease or diabetes. Men more than 20% overweight are one and a half times more likely to die prematurely.

— One-fifth of Americans are so overweight that their health is threatened (according to Theodore Cooper, former Assistant Secretary of Health, Education and Welfare, in testimony before the United States Senate).

— According to one government poll taken in recent years, 9.5 million Americans said they were on a diet, 16.4 million were watching their weight so they wouldn't gain, and 26.1 million expressed concern about how much they weighed.

Obviously, Americans are concerned about their weight. There are still, however, many myths about food that some of us continue to believe in as we attempt to get to our desired weight. Here are some of the food fallacies collected by the American Diabetes Association:

— Fad diets really do work, and if not, you can always get double your money back.

— Toast has fewer calories than bread.

— Margarine contains fewer calories than butter.

— Obesity is due mostly to heredity.

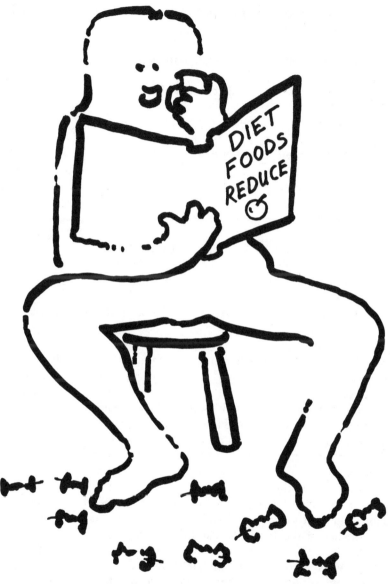

There are, however, many myths about food that
some of us continue to believe in.

— You can eat all you want and still lose weight if you take the right "reducing pill."

— Gelatin desserts are nonfattening.

— Eating grapefruit will cause weight loss.

— For some people, all food turns to fat.

— High-protein foods are low in calories.

— Fruits are low in calories.

— Skipping a meal is a good way to lose weight.

— Sugar is not as fattening as starch.

— Honey has fewer calories than sugar.

— "De-starched" potato chips do not have many calories.

It is amazing how gullible we can be when it comes to eating. We kid ourselves that the calories that we get by licking the spoon don't count, or that the food we eat between meals really isn't *that* fattening. We want so much to "have our cake and eat it too" that we actually talk ourselves into believing misinformation like that listed above. Face it: The only thing that happens to a piece of bread when it is toasted is that a few molecules of water evaporate from it — and we all know how many calories that saves us!

It's obvious then, that we, as a nation of fat people, need to start paying closer attention to our nutritional needs on a realistic basis: one that doesn't fool with facts; one that takes into account the quality of the foods we eat (fiber versus fat, unprocessed versus processed foods) as well as the *quantity* (calories) we take in. This means cutting down on all those flab-making fats, sluggish sugars, and sinister salts that characterize the fast foods and processed goodies we constantly see, read, and hear about through the media. Instead of weighing down our bodies and brains with such noxious "nutrients," we need to increase the proportion of fiber in our diets and eat unprocessed foods rich in the vitamins, minerals and lean proteins we really need to perform at our best and to enjoy our lives to the fullest (not the "fillest").

There are many good nutritional plans available in this era of growing health consciousness. Over the past several years, our increasing concern with nutritional health has yielded an ava-lanche of books and organizations dedicated to educating us about our food needs. So I won't bore you here with another nutritional plan (although, in Appendix II of this book you will find a list of basic nutrients and the foods that provide them, along with a list of recommended publications and organizations for further information). Most of us — especially those of us who have battled the bulge for years — are already aware that certain foods (such as lean fish broiled without oil) are better for us than others (prime rib slavered with butter — fat on fat). The chal-lenge that obese people face is usually not that they don't *know* what isn't good for them but, rather, that they haven't built up strategies for avoiding "bad" foods and eating appropriate amounts of good foods. Here, then, are some basic guidelines for eating better as a matter of habit.

GROCERIES *vs* GROSSERIES

In this day of high restaurant prices and low budgets, most of us (unless we live on a farm) are meeting our nutritional needs by purchasing our food at the market and preparing it at home. This is especially true for those of us with families: When three, four, or more of us go out to eat, those fast (and fattening) foods are often all we can afford. But whether it's just you and your cat or you and a family of ten, preparing your own food is your best route to well-balanced and modest-sized meals. (Never fear, you single eat-outers, I'll get to you in a minute!)

The first step is to get the food, right? And where do you get it? At the grocery store, and that's not spelled g-r-o-s-s-e-r-i-e, although it could be if you let it. Supermarkets are often more dangerous than the latest TV commercial that offers two-for-the-price-of-one pizza dripping with cheese. At the supermarket, boxes upon cartons of sugar-laden, fat-infested processed foods, attractively packaged and on sale for half price, are right there, within reach, waiting for hungry eyes and outsized appetites to stash them in the shopping cart.

The first rule of grocery shopping, then, is **never shop when you are hungry.** If you have to shop on the way home from work, right before dinner (as many of us do), be sure to swallow a glass of skim milk or eat a piece of fruit beforehand (and don't forget to skip the milk or fruit during dinner).

Rule two is to **plan ahead.** Have your list of necessary foods in hand as you wheel down the supermarket lanes — and don't swerve from the items on your list, or the area of the store in which you will find them (unless, of course, you have to swerve for an oncoming cart!).

Speaking of locations in the store: You will find the most nutritious (unprocessed) foods on the outer perimeter of the store. That's where you will see the fruits and vegetables, dairy products (again, stick to the skim milk and the plain yoghurt), fish, poultry, and freshly baked breads. The canned and processed foods are stored in the center aisles, along with the snack foods and your everyday "junk food." Oh, there are some healthy foods in the center, such as pasta, beans, and legumes — as well as those nonfood items such as dishwashing liquid and toilet paper — but most of the foods you *need* to eat are located on the outer edges of the market.

Okay, you've been to the market and have purchased only those items you really need. Now you're at home, unpacking them. The question here is, To freeze or not to freeze? Whether you are single or have a large family, if you have planned your shopping well you know just what you will need to prepare within the next few days and what will need to be stored for a week or two. Invest in a box of freezer bags and meal-size plastic containers and **store the food you have purchased in meal-size servings.** For example, open that package of chicken legs and place one or two (for a single meal) or four to six (for a family meal) in a freezer bag. When you defrost the chicken next week, you won't run the risk of preparing a meal that promises lots of leftovers and plenty of temptation for you.

When preparing a serving size, remember that about three-quarters to one cup is plenty for a single helping. The size of your fist is a good, healthy serving of food. A piece of meat about the size of your palm is about three to four ounces. A chicken thigh or drumstick contains about two ounces of meat, a wing about one ounce, and a breast about three ounces. A one-inch cube or one-quarter cup of cheese is about one ounce. If you eat two fist-size servings of food per meal (say, one of fish and the other of a vegetable), you have filled your stomach to capacity.

Okay, meal's over. If you've handled this well, you are physically satisfied and not uncomfortable (not "stuffed"), and there are no leftovers, since you prepared meal-size portions rather than a five-day casserole. "What?" I hear you moaning, "You mean I have to cook for this demanding family every night? The last thing I need is to be around food more often!"

Alright, then. I can certainly see that. Besides, who wants to cook five (or even two) nights in a row when you were planning to go to your weaving class (or your group session) tomorrow night? So here's another tip: **When you do have leftovers, don't put them away IN you, put them away FROM you.** Freeze that casserole for next week's evening activity. If you leave it in its chewable state, you may find yourself chewing off more than you or your desired weight can handle.

EATING OUT

Eating out is hard to avoid, but it does have its advantages. That is, you are around food less often — no preparation and no packing away of leftovers. The disadvantages, however, can cancel these out: Restaurant portions are twice the size they need to be, and restaurant food usually comes packed with all the fats, salts, and sugars that make the affluent diet such a disaster for good health. On top of all that, all those social tapes playing in our heads (see Chapter 4) are twice as hard to buck when we eat out. Here are some of them:

"I'm paying for it, so I might as well get what I pay for." This thinking can be changed to *"I'll eat as much as I need now and take the rest home in a people bag."*

"I deserve to treat myself to dinner out. I've worked all day, and I'm pooped." This needs to be changed to *"I deserve a treat for my aching body. I'll take a hot bath and read a chapter from my new book before dinner."*

"I can't waste this food here at the restaurant. It's so good, and I can always diet tomorrow." Change this to *"WASTE or WAIST?"*

Here are some ways to survive eating out:

Again, **plan ahead.** Pick a place with a varied and healthy menu so you'll at least get some good nutrition along with your calories. A list of restaurants that will prepare delicious food that is low in fat and cholesterol and will otherwise accommodate those who have dietary restrictions is available from the American Heart Association. The pamphlet may be obtained by contacting your local AHA chapter.

Decide before you enter the restaurant how many calories you will "splurge" on, and then STICK TO IT.

Feel virtuous when others break down and order a hot fudge sundae while you choose to pass. Stick to your resolve!

Expect that you will be taking food home with you, since those restaurant portions are so oversized, and pat yourself on the back for getting two meals for the price of one! If you feel comfortable, share one dinner with a friend and order a separate dinner salad — without dressing. You can add your own low-calorie preparation (many delicious ones are available in the market) and save as much as 500 calories per ladle.

Dealing with the menu: For the first course, try fruit, juice, or consomme. As for entrees, remember the "four B's": bake, broil, boil, and barbeque (no sauce, please). All fried foods, including fried zucchini and other "low-calorie" fried veggies), are fattening. Cream sauces and gravies are fattening. If you eat steak, eat filet mignon, flank, or sirloin, which have less fat than prime rib and other marbled beef. Side dishes should be sauceless — try sliced tomatoes without the vinaigrette, asparagus without the Hollandaise sauce, or a plain baked potato (only about a hundred calories without butter or sour cream). Again, you can take along your own condiments — butter substitute (the kind that comes as a powder) and mixed herbs — or request plain vinegar or lemon slices. For dessert, savor a good cup of coffee or tea, or order fruit. If your dinner companion is willing, you can take a taste of his or her dessert. A taste will satisfy your taste buds, and if you have eaten slowly (which is often easier to do in a restaurant than at home), you will notice that you aren't really hungry for more food anyway. The feeling of walking away from a restaurant without an immediate need to grab the bicarbonate of soda is a great one!

PLAN AHEAD, FOLLOW THROUGH

These, then, are a few strategies for dealing with your eating day. Remember, *weight is in consciousness,* which means that your eating behavior every day must be in your consciousness — right up there with your agenda for work meetings and taking the kids to their swimming lessons. *Plan ahead:* List your dietary needs in consultation with your family physician and with the aid of the information given in Appendix II. Then *follow through.* Stick to your resolve! And to help yourself do so, continue your daily ten minutes of Reflective Relearning, focusing on your planned eating behavior for the day. As you continue to follow constructive courses of action in relation to food, your newfound strategies will become ingrained in your right brain and subconscious mind. You will begin to find yourself "on your right weigh" — for life!

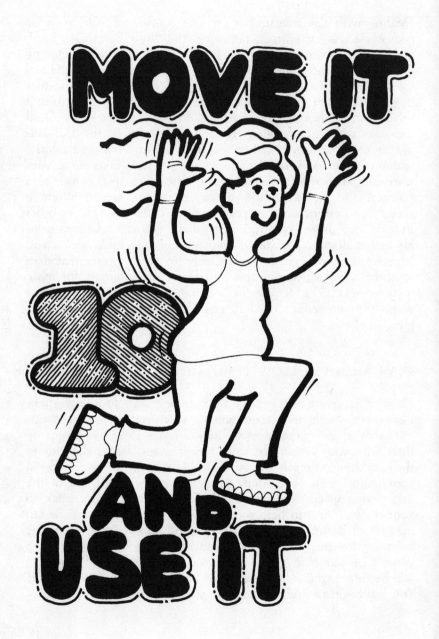

THIS CHAPTER IS ABOUT THE VALUE of an increased activity level in obtaining, maintaining, and sustaining your desired weight. We will discuss several types of activities suitable for assisting you in achieving this goal — exercises you can do right now. It is important, before starting any new exercise program, that you consult your physician and pay close attention to the section in this chapter called SAFETY FIRST.

Throughout this book, I have hammered at the idea that "losing" weight is a faulty premise. The ideal of weight loss is what keeps many people fat as they become trapped in the gain-loss merry-go-round.

Actually, we can never truly "lose" anything. We may move it around, but we never lose it. Modern physics has demonstrated that the universe is a self-contained whole. There are no leaks. The popularization of recycling is based on this fact: We recycle our newspapers, our aluminum cans, our old clothes, our reparable toys and furniture, even our water. When we exercise, then, we recycle the energy that is currently manifesting itself as fat around our hips. That recycled fat energy becomes other kinds of energy, through creativity and action. For example, the energy we have been expending on eating, we can expend on being politically active or taking a class or even shopping for new clothes (since our old ones don't fit anymore, and we recycled them to Goodwill or the Salvation Army).

Remember, the direction of the world is from thought to action to form. Everything that exists in this world is a product of this process. First we review our thought patterns concerning food: We become *aware* that we are "eating this and feeling better." Next, we take action: We find an appropriate exercise place, one with people who also have a weight challenge. Finally, we experience our new form: a body that is what we want it to be.

The entire world is holistic. We never lose anything — but we can change it to another, more desirable, form. We recycle energy when we walk or jog or dance or row. We move our bodies, and the energy that has expressed itself in fat moves off our bodies and into the atmosphere. Physiologically, we become more energetic as we become more fit. This new energy is obviously recycled from our fat.

Now we consciously *choose* to look at our thought patterns, uncovering the hidden agenda behind our compulsive eating habits. Next, we take conscious, deliberate action by noticing our behavior but not blaming or punishing ourselves. Instead, we build a better plan. We can, for example, choose, deliberately, to put down that cookie and get dressed for our exercise class. Gradually, a new form begins to appear. Not by magic, of course, or by external environmental intervention, but through our conscious decisions about what we've done in the past and what we consciously decide to do today.

Our second step consists of *taking action*. The action we need to take is basically twofold. First, we must begin the inner process of visualization, or Reflective Relearning, which was described in detail in Chapters 6, 7, and 8. Second, we must begin to increase our level of activity. Physical activity allows us to recycle some of our fat into another form of energy. We're not going to lose this energy. We can't. But we can reprocess it from stored fat energy into energy for positive uses, through exercise.

EXERCISE: PAIN OR PLEASURE?

Whenever the word "exercise" is mentioned, many of us blanch and grow weak. In our culture, exercise has been linked to punishment. How often do we think of doing pushups or taking the proverbial laps around a track as a form of punishment? I recall a story about a man who was quite obese as a child. His classmates and he were often told to do laps, and, of course, he was always the last one to finish running. The coach would make the other students run an extra lap so that they would finish at about the same time as this obese youngster. You can imagine the razzing he took afterward in the locker room. No wonder so many fat people hate the thought of exercising! Many still remember horrid experiences of this sort from their P.E. classes.

Fat children, especially girls, loathe having to undress in front of "normal" kids. They endure terrible insults, wounds that make indelible marks on their minds and feelings. Exercise is forever associated in their minds with embarrassment, ridicule, and harassment.

What we all need to learn is that exercise is pleasant. Increased physical activity can be fun. Today, we can participate in all kinds of exercise classes. They can be exciting, social, and stimulating. There are adult classes in tap dancing, belly dancing, clogging, slimnastics — you name it, and someone teaches it. It is really possible for you to break out of your old, negative associations of having to sweat and be humiliated in front of others because you were fat and awkward.

It may be an old saw that "the fat lady is light on her feet," but it is often true that many overweight people have great timing. Obese people are often more skillful and graceful on their feet than many of their nonobese friends — when they allow themselves to participate in dance and other physical exercise. Health spas and gyms are becoming more sensitive to the special needs of the obese client and now offer separate classes for people who are twenty or more pounds overweight. You don't have to walk into an exercise class wearing a size XXL leotard and have to compare yourself to an Olive Oyl in a size 3 complaining that she just *has* to lose that extra tenth of a pound. People who don't have to compare themselves with the local Twiggies are more likely to stay in their exercise classes — and to succeed. Check your own neighborhood for special classes in exercise for people who are at least twenty pounds overweight.

GETTING STARTED: TIPS AND TABOOS

If you've read Chapter 4, you're highly aware that our society feeds us skinny messages with every television commercial. Every women's magazine is full of ways to be thin — from diet fads to the latest way to exercise to ways to get the fat to roll off our bodies by using marvelous new machines. Well, I've said a lot about the reasons that diets don't work. Here, I want to talk a bit about "exercise hype": Let the buyer beware!

We see a lot of ads these days for health spas and exercise machines. They urge us to buy bicycles that go nowhere except in front of the television set and rebounders for those rainy days when we can't get out and jog. We have European health spas with the latest fancy equipment that, we are told, keeps all of the beautiful people in Paris very thin and desirable. We have special jump ropes that cost a bunch of money to keep in our bedrooms so we can jump while we watch TV and brush our teeth at the same time. We are bombarded with messages to *squeeze in* that exercise time, no matter what.

I happen to be big on exercise, so I'm sure not knocking it. What I am knocking is the emphasis on gadgetry, on instantaneous rewards. I'm questioning the hard-sell that keeps us on the lookout for a new gadget to buy next to melt the fat from those thighs.

We have allowed ourselves to be exploited. We join expensive gyms because we receive a tremendous discount if we join for the whole year right now. Get it while it's hot! We all seem to be lured by this idea of joining up for a year because it's so cheap. Often, when people calculate at the end of the year how much they actually spent per session for the times they attended, they are appalled. Sure, health spas work. They work just fine — as long as we GO THERE AND WORK OUT. But enthusiasm soon dwindles, muscles get sore, and we get busy.

Boy, do we get busy. Can't possibly find time to go to workouts, what with Girl Scouts, our jobs, commuting, meetings, practice every night, grocery shopping, taking the cat to the vet, getting our hair permed . . . . So we exercise our jaws a lot to our friends about how we intend to get back on the track just as soon as the kids go back to school in the fall, or just as soon as they are out of school for the summer, or just after the holidays. This type of reasoning is first cousin to the rationalizations we use for postponing proper eating. We buy the hype, and we do it with great faith and excellent intentions. But, as my grandmother used to say, the road paved with good intentions sure doesn't lead to heaven.

The point is this: Because we are a nation of guilt-ridden fat people, we fall for the hype and join spas before we give ourselves a fair shake to see if we will stick to a program for even one week, let alone a whole year. Working on the old dictate of "waste not, want not," we buy the "large economy size" and use less than half of it.

And we're into exercise clothes. We buy expensive jogging suits that cost more than Mother paid for her entire wedding ensemble, only to find that those fancy sweats are really too warm to jog in. We learn to buy special shoes for jogging, tennis, racketball, and dance class. Sure, if we decide that jogging is our thing, then it is best to go out and buy the proper shoes. First, however, we need to do a little testing. We need to go on regular walk-jogs in our old tennies to see if we will stick to it for even one week. If we do, it makes sense to invest in running shoes that will protect our feet — but not until we've made that commitment.

The obvious point here is that a lot of us leap — and only then remember that we didn't look first. We have great intentions because of the cultural prompting to look good. We really do want to fit in and be as skinny as Mary at the bridge club or Barbie at the spa. But before you and I run out and buy all the latest trappings of a particular exercise or sport or health club, we need to be sure that we'll stick with it long enough for the investment to pay off.

Many people get depressed with this cycle of becoming enthusiastic about a new exercise place or the latest do-it-yourself exercise kit, then investing, then losing interest. Or they become angry. Both of these are emotional cues that lead them back toward food. I urge you to start by seeking out inexpensive places to exercise. Many colleges, YMCAs, and other community facilities offer low-cost beginners' classes. If you find that you attend fairly regularly for a month or more, you may wish to join a fancier club or spa. But first see if you will stay on a program for just three times a week for just one month. If you commit yourself to twelve sessions, you are likely to go on working out weekly.

Encourage some of your friends or neighbors to meet you for morning or after-dinner walks. When this becomes routine for you, then go out and buy that neat warm-up suit and good shoes, because you'll use them. Otherwise, someone else will be buying them from the church bazaar a few years from now brand-new.

PUTTING YOUR HEART IN IT: AEROBICS

Aerobic exercise is generally viewed by physicians as an essential form of exercise. The word aerobic comes from the word "aerobe,"

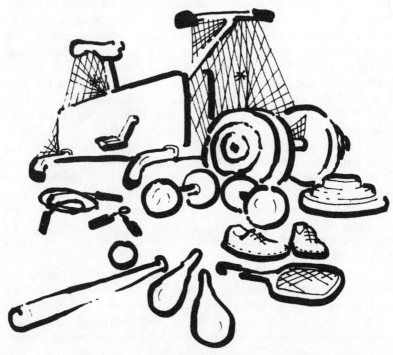

Before buying all the latest trappings of an exercise or sport we need to be sure that we'll stick with it.

which is an organism that requires oxygen or air to live. The root word, *aero* (air), is combined with the Greek word *bios* (life) to make the word aerobic.

Covert Bailey, author of *Fit or Fat?*, defines aerobic exercise as steady, uninterrupted exercise at 80% of your maximum recommended training heart rate (see MONITORING YOUR PULSE RATE, below) sustained for twelve minutes. For most of us, work is not exercise, because it does not entail such physical exertion or, if it does, that exercise is rarely sustained for twelve minutes at 80% of the maximum training heart rate. Indeed, for many of us, our work is sedentary — few of us ever have to "huff and puff" on the job.

It's the huffing and puffing (aerobic exercise) that strengthens the body's oxygen delivery system. Air is taken into the lungs, where it is diffused in the blood and pumped by the heart throughout the body via arteries and capillaries, which transport the oxygen-carrying red blood cells to every other cell in the body. This nourishment of the cells keeps our bodies alive. With aerobic exercise, we obtain, maintain, and sustain physical fitness, which means that the body is better able to use the nutritious oxygen it takes in.

Aerobic exercise plus good nutrition prevents the formation of "sludge" in the arteries. Sludge is the clumping together of red blood cells — the oxygen-carrying ones — and is much less efficient than individually traveling cells. It also leads to blockage of the blood vessels, which may be fatal. Aerobic exercise plus good nutrition creates the long, slim, strong muscles that are aesthetically pleasing. It's their muscles that make ballerinas, for example, look so good.

Since few of us work as ballerinas or athletes, we must look to activities other than our work in order to stay fit. Spot-reducing exercises, though popular, do not exercise our heart muscles sufficiently to use the energy we have poured into our bodies as calories. Bouncing your butt on the floor is like tenderizing a Swiss steak. Let's face it: We can't bump it off, beat it off, roll it off, or wish it off. Fat simply will not leave unless we do aerobics to recycle the energy off our hips. We can do exercises such as situps or leg lifts to *tone* individual muscle groups, and toning is important for good looks. Yet, without adding the aerobic workout that actually burns fat, we may end up with toned muscles under a layer of fat.

Here are some of the more familiar aerobic exercises:

Outdoor Aerobics

Jogging and running are the best-known aerobic exercises. As a rule of thumb, if you take more than eight minutes to cover a mile, you're jogging. Before you embark on any jogging or running program, consult your physician and seek counsel from an exercise physiologist if possible. Buy the proper shoes (again, consult an exercise physiologist), and run on proper surfaces, such as dirt or sand. *Never* run on concrete. And remember, not everyone is a jogger/runner. There are other ways of doing aerobic exercise, including . . .

Power-walking. This is an excellent aerobic exercise for people of all ages — particularly if you are overweight or just out of shape. It takes most people about twenty minutes to walk one mile. "Power-walking" means that you walk as quickly as you comfortably can, swinging your arms, to get your pulse rate up (we will cover pulse rates later in this chapter). If this doesn't get your pulse rate high enough, you can carry weights in your hands or in a backpack.

Cycling is good for people who are extremely overweight, as it is less taxing on the legs and back. You may have to go far to find safe places to ride, where there is less stop and go, but the exhilaration of covering miles of beautiful countryside is worth it.

Swimming is good for your heart and lungs and for limbering up all the muscles. To make it aerobic, however, you must really plow the water. Leisurely crawlers will find swimming less effective than running, jogging, or power-walking for reducing fat. Remember, whales and seals are not particularly slim!

Cross-country skiing is an excellent aerobic exercise, as it works all the muscles. It is a godsend if you live in a region where snow would otherwise leave you housebound for several months of the year.

Roller-skating and **ice-skating** provide the benefits of running without many of the attendant problems (such as pounding feet and stressing knees). Again, as with swimming, one must put in some effort and keep going to realize maximum benefit.

Indoor Aerobics

Jumping rope is a good aerobic exercise. Make sure that the surface on which you jump is soft and that the rope is the right length. The handles should reach your nipples when you stand on the center of the rope with both feet. Jump with alternate feet at about seventy jumps per minute.

Running in place is another good aerobic exercise. Be sure to lift your legs as high as you can. A fit person may need to lift his knees very high; an unfit person can derive benefit by lifting the knees to a lower level.

The stationary bicycle is good for unfit, older, or overweight persons. Be sure that you buy a good, sturdy one — preferably without a motor!

Rowing machines require an expensive investment, but when used properly they exercise nearly all the major muscles of your body.

A treadmill must be paced at a fast walk or a very slow jog for twelve minutes or more to be effective. Again, there is quite an outlay of money at the beginning.

Jumping jacks are very strenuous but also very effective. Many experts recommend that you do these every other day, with less traumatic exercises in between.

Dancing is very popular and has the added advantage of music, which stimulates the right brain. It is recommended that you keep dancing for twelve minutes to realize the aerobic benefits. No stops for beverages!

A mini-trampoline or rebounder is an excellent source of aerobic exercise, with minimum trauma to the body. You can dance on it, run on it, walk on it, or just bounce.

According to Marilyn Grant, Director of Dancerobics in Whittier, California, some specific physical changes can result from regular aerobic exercise:

— You breathe easier, as the muscles in your chest wall become stronger.

— Your heart beats more strongly. More blood is pumped with each stroke, thereby distributing oxygen more rapidly throughout the body.

— Your blood vessels increase in size and number, thus enriching tissues with more oxygen for more energy.

— You have better blood circulation and lowered blood pressure.

— Your muscles become much stronger.

— After aerobic exercise, you have a feeling of released tension. This leads to a sense of relaxation.

Most people aim for at least twelve minutes of sustained aerobics in the beginning and work toward twenty to thirty minutes when they get into good shape. The heart is a big muscle. Sustained, vigorous exercise strengthens the heart, and it needn't work as hard to do the same amount of work. A fit heart has fewer beats, but at the same time it pumps more blood with each contraction, thereby distributing oxygen more rapidly throughout the body. After aerobic exercise, you feel more alive, because your body is conserving energy.

MONITORING YOUR PULSE RATE

You should monitor your heart by checking your pulse rate after each aerobic session of sustained intensity. If your pulse rate is too high, you are overexerting yourself and building up chronic exhaustion. If the pulse rate is too low, you are not going to make any measurable changes in your body. If you plan to exercise regularly, it is vital to your health and well-being that you understand and follow the information below, as well as consult your physician before starting any exercise program.

In order to measure your heart rate accurately, you need to know the different heart rate definitions. The **resting heart rate** may be calculated by taking your pulse three mornings in a row. You can take your pulse at your carotid artery, which is in the front strip of muscle running vertically in your neck. Use the tips of your three middle fingers. One of these fingers will pick up the pulse. Do not use your thumb, as it has its own strong pulse. You can also take your pulse inside your wrist, although this is more difficult for beginners to feel. Then you simply count the beats for one minute.

The average resting heart rate for women is 78 to 84 beats per minute; for men, it is 72 to 78. Once you have taken your rate for three mornings in a row, average them out to get your average resting heart rate.

The next rates you will want to measure are your **training heart rate** and your **recommended training heart rate.** You can find your training heart rate by counting your beats during activity for ten seconds and multiplying by six, or by counting your heart rate for six seconds and multiplying by ten. You should do this after each 12 minute session of aerobic activity. If you are receiving the full benefit of your exercise, your heart rate will register between 60 and 80 percent of its maximum output, which is around 220 beats per minute. Therefore, the formula used to determine your recommended training heart rate (THR) is based on this number (220) minus your age, and multiplied by the percentage of output you want to achieve. For example, if you are 45 years old, and wish to work at 60 percent of your maximum heart rate, your formula would look like this:

220 − 45 (age) = 175 x .60 (percentage)
= 105 (recommended THR)

Or you could choose to work at 80% of your maximum heart

rate, which would be a real aerobic workout. In that case your formula would be:

$$220 - 45 = 175 \times .80 \text{ (percentage)}$$
$$= 140 \text{ (recommended THR)}$$

The average training heart rate varies widely for different individuals.

The **recovery heart rate** is next. This is measured five minutes after a cool-down exercise, which is one that gradually slows the pace until you are moving rather slowly. After five minutes have elapsed and you have completed the cool-down exercise, count your heartbeat for fifteen seconds and multiply by four. Your recovery heart rate should be 120 beats per minute or less. A ten-minute recovery rate should be below 100 beats per minute, or twenty-five beats per fifteen seconds.

The more fit you are, the faster your heart rate returns to normal. If your recovery rate is too high, you need to dance or exercise at a lower level the next time. When you exercise regularly (at least three times a week), you should see your heart rate start to return to normal more quickly.

SAFETY FIRST

Many obese people are concerned about how safe aerobic exercise is. According to experts, any form of exercise, including aerobics, contains an element of risk. A study conducted by the National Injury Prevention Foundation of San Diego, California, recently found that 76.3% of 200 aerobic dance instructors incurred or aggravated an injury while conducting their classes. Most of these injuries were to the legs, feet, ankles, or back. This is what the instructors are suffering, so we can only guess at what the novice is up against.

Here are a few safety tips for you to consider while doing aerobic exercises:

1. When you are thinking of embarking on an aerobic exercise

program, remember that it is important to consult your physician to make sure your heart and lungs and other important organs are in shape to take the level of exercise intended.

2. When equipment is required, be sure you get the proper kind, whether it be running shoes, jogging bras, weights, or a sturdy rebounder. Special aerobic exercise shoes can help prevent injuries. Do not wear your running shoes to aerobics classes. Running shoes are designed to increase traction, and when you are dancing or moving from side to side, increased traction is the last thing you want. The court shoes you wear for tennis or racquetball are better than running shoes for dance or exercise classes. These are designed to slide as you change directions. They also give better side-to-side support than most running shoes. If you decide to buy special aerobic shoes, be sure you've been in the class long enough to know you'll stick with it. Then make sure these shoes provide adequate support and have good side-to-side stability, good impact cushioning, and a surface that will slide along the floor.

3. Be sure you are warmed up and stretched out before you begin to exercise. Place your mind in the muscle group with which you are working. It is important that you "think into" that group of muscles in order to allow them to relax.

4. Do not attempt to keep up with seasoned exercisers, especially the instructor. Enter jumping exercises, for example, very slowly. Strenuous jumping can put as much as two to three times the force of your body weight on your feet. Therefore, if you are very overweight, jump in moderation. Go at your own pace. Compliment yourself on your private accomplishments.

5. While exercising, wear shorts and a T-shirt or a leotard and exercise hosiery (tights). Do not wear rubber or plastic suits to exercise. The body is a natural air conditioner: It responds to physical exertion with perspiration, which has to evaporate for the body to cool off. Restrictive clothing drives the body temperature too high, and when this occurs, you will lose water, not fat.

6. When working out with a regular routine, be sure to drink when you are thirsty. There is no restriction on your water intake, although you should avoid gulping down huge amounts at once and risking cramps. Listen to your body. It will tell you how much you need. And stop exercising if you feel any pain — pressure is okay, but no pain. Let your lungs breathe normally. No need to exaggerate the huffing and puffing.

7. A safety precaution for women: Do situps in a bent-knee position, and always curl the back as you come up. Women who do straight-leg situps tend to injure themselves. When doing lateral leg lifts (on your side), make sure your hip does not rotate outward. Keep the side of your leg facing the ceiling; otherwise, the front muscles (quadriceps) take over, and you are not exercising the muscles for which lateral leg lifts are designed.

Aerobics will burn up many more calories than floorwork will. After an aerobic workout, you body continues to burn calories at a high rate for three to four hours. But take care not to get overenthusiastic at first: When you are working in your "red zone" (heart rate too fast), you are not only exhausting yourself, you are burning sugar. Working at your safe rate (70 – 80% of your training heart rate) burns fat, which is what you want to burn. Go for the long, slower distances for more lasting, safer results.

Remember, fitness is not stored, but fat is! Every forty-eight to seventy-two hours, you need to work out to maintain adult fitness. Doing aerobic exercises only two days a week means you need additional workouts. Variety is good, so consider swimming, jogging, or bicycling on the days you do not do other aerobic exercises. Whatever you choose to do, do it at least three times a week, for twelve minutes each time. Thirty-six minutes a week is not much to ask for the feeling of well-being and the FUN you'll get in exchange. It's quite a bargain!

PE: FROM PANIC EXPERIENCE
TO POWER EDUCATION

Before ending this chapter, I'd like to share with you the experiences of a woman with whom I worked not long ago. To protect her identity, I'll call her Darlene.

Darlene was born with a congenital hip problem which is not uncommon in children. Today, pediatricians often identify and correct this problem in infancy. Darlene, however, was born in the early 1930s, when little was known about the corrective measures. Consequently, her condition was never identified, and, as she grew up, one of her legs turned in. Her family chalked it up to her being pigeon-toed. As Darlene grew, her condition became a terrible problem, as she was continually tripping over her feet. When she was about 14, her parents divorced, and she began a rapid weight gain. As she grew heavier, the foot-tripping became worse. She tried to be excused from her physical education classes in school, but her doctor merely told her to be more careful and try not to trip. (Unfortunately, the attitude toward her condition in the 1930s and 1940s was not as sophisticated as it is today.)

By the time Darlene was in high school gym class, she weighed thirty pounds more than her desired weight and was as clumsy as the proverbial ox. She was an outstanding student in all of her academic classes, but she began to fail P.E. Of course, she could not graduate until she had completed her P.E. requirements. In those days, school counseling was virtually unheard of, and her mother was too absorbed in personal problems to be of any help.

Darlene realized that she had to get through her P.E. classes no matter how painful it was for her psychologically. She desperately wanted to graduate, and she literally forced herself to attend gym class. The week the class had final exams, part of the test was to compete in a relay race. This relay consisted of running a certain distance, going over a hurdle, and climbing a rope as part of a team. Naturally, when her teacher placed her on a team, Darlene's teammates let loose with moans and groans. As you might imagine, Darlene was a mass of jelly. Her anxiety level was so high that when it was her turn to compete, she was doomed before she left the bench. Even if she hadn't been thirty pounds overweight and even if she hadn't had an undiagnosed congenital hip rotation, her anxiety alone would have done her in.

She did terribly. The crowning blow came when she finally got to the rope at the end of the relay: she was so out of breath and so miserably embarrassed that she could not complete the climb. The entire class stood and watched as she struggled over and over to get to the top, only to slide back down. Her team-mates booed her, and some of them even cried, because she caused their team to lose. The teacher finally had the mercy to call her down and disqualify the team.

Darlene never bothered to shower or go to her locker to get her street clothes. She ran to a nearby wooded area and huddled under the shrubs for the entire afternoon and night. Her mother finally called the police to look for her. When they found her at ten the next morning, she was in a terrible state, almost inco-herent, and babbling that she was a failure and wanted to die. The police took her home. She was very tired but unable to sleep. She stayed in her room for two more days, neither eating nor sleeping. Finally, she decided to kill herself, and jumped from the balcony of her three-story home. Although she didn't die, she did break several bones and sustained a concussion.

Darlene was subsequently placed in a "mental ward," as it was called then, and received some psychotherapy after her release from the hospital. However, she and her mother were unable to pay for further assistance, and she was released within two weeks of her admission to the "mental ward." She flatly refused to return to school and dropped out. She worked in a dime store for two years and then moved into sales work in a department store where she remained for the next twenty-four years, working her way up to assistant buyer in household appliances.

During those years, Darlene took many adult education cour-ses but never applied for college credit. She was careful not to let anyone know that she had never graduated from high school. Since she was so bright, well-read, and educated in her own right, she pulled it off very well. She never married, throwing herself into her work one hundred percent instead. When she and I first met, she weighed in excess of 200 pounds. I met her at a weight clinic, where she was making her first serious attempt to "lose weight."

In the group, it became apparent to me that she was self-taught and very intelligent. After we had been friends for about six months and I had worked with her in the weight group, I approached her after one session and suggested that we talk for a while. We stood in the parking lot for at least four hours while she began to express her concerns. She was miserable and terribly frightened that others would discover that she had failed to graduate from high school.

Darlene subsequently made an appointment with me, and we began individual psychotherapy. During the following year, she learned so much about herself that it was incredible. When she learned about her hip, she was astounded. She then understood where her "clumsiness" came from. She went to an orthopedic medical doctor and began as much remediation for her condition as was possible. Of course, she could not be totally restored, but there were some things that she could do. She wore special shoes and did some exercises to help correct her condition. Interestingly enough, Darlene had never considered sitting for the examination in her state that would grant her a high school diploma. She had been so thoroughly traumatized by the P.E. experience that she could not face going back to "climb" that "rope."

Incredible as this story may sound, it is not uncommon. When a person undergoes something so terrifying that he or she attempts suicide, the trauma can last for years.

Nevertheless, Darlene finally did decide to take the examination, and she was delighted to see how easy it was. She passed with flying colors, and was utterly thrilled that she had finally received her diploma. She subsequently enrolled in a retail-marketing class in a community college and she plans to go right through until she has a college degree — a dream long forgone but now within reach.

In terms of exercise, the hardest part for Darlene to face was the episode of the relay race. We spent hours in progressive Reflective Relearning to help her overcome the horror of that day. Although her suicide attempt and the resultant broken bones had little physical impact on her, the emotional scars did not fade. Gradually, she began at least to talk about doing some exercises. She agreed to meet with me one hour before the regular group session to go for a walk. She was amazed that her new shoes and the special lifts in them assisted her in walking straighter than she thought possible. Soon, she agreed to observe a slimnastics class with a friend. The teacher was very understanding, allowing Darlene simply to stand at the back of the room. Then, ever so slowly, Darlene gathered her courage and began to participate.

Today, Darlene is still about forty pounds overweight, but that is sixty pounds lighter than she was when she began. She sticks to appropriate, moderate exercises and is considering the possibility of wearing a leotard when she is another ten pounds closer to her desired weight.

LET'S GET PHYSICAL

Like other individuals whose stories I have shared with you, Darlene was so excited about her progress that she wanted to share her experience with everyone. She realized that not everyone can afford a year of individual psychotherapy, so she asked me to share with you her experience in the hope that others could see that they are not alone and perhaps, as a result, learn to face their greatest fears. If Darlene could confront her fear after her extreme trauma, surely there are many among you who, perhaps having undergone less threatening experiences, can meet the challenge of entering an exercise program.

It is my hope that you will decide, on your own, to do so. When you do, it is imperative that you study the personality of the exercise instructor (if you chose to take a class). The teacher needs to be aware of the special challenges the overweight person faces — and, as I have said earlier in this chapter, there are an increasing number of communities that offer special exercise classes designed for those who are overweight or just entering an exercise program after a long period of inactivity. Seek them out and, if possible, attend with a friend. The moral support you can gain from a friend who is also overweight is particularly rewarding, for you have the added satisfaction of knowing that you are providing, as well as receiving, that support.

In this sedentary age too many of us — overweight or not — have forgotten (or simply repressed) how much satisfaction and fun we can get from exercising and feeling one with our bodies. Remember, it is your right to participate fully in any physical activity in which you have an interest. Stop thinking that you are "unathletic" or "not physical." You will be surprised at how a little physical activity can yield monumentally positive emotional and mental results. Approach your entry into physical exercise slowly and with conviction, and you, like Darlene, will learn to "move it and use it" — and have a lot of fun in the process!

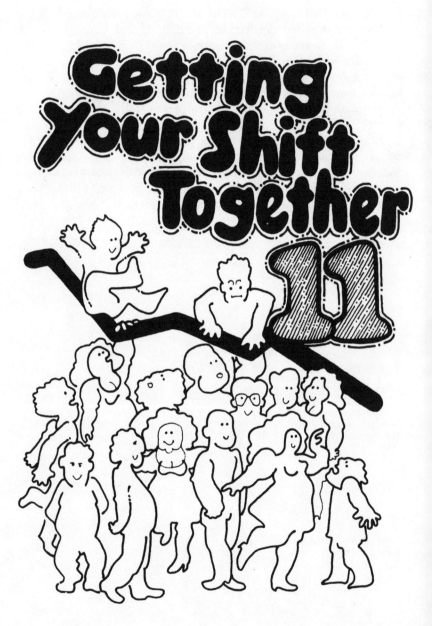

IN THIS BOOK, WE HAVE TAKEN A JOURNEY — a journey through the mind and brain — and have moved from the old, subconscious attitudes of "eat this and feel better" to a new awareness of our eating patterns. This awareness allows us to make conscious decisions about food and about all those activities (from confronting our emotions directly to exercising our bodies) that we have allowed food to replace. If you have adhered faithfully to the six-week introductory program of Reflective Relearning that was outlined in Chapter 8, and have incorporated into your daily routine at least a few of the suggestions for dealing with food and exercise presented in Chapters 9 and 10, you are "on your right weigh."

In fact, once you have made this commitment to recognizing old right-brain, subconscious behaviors and to reprogramming them through Reflective Relearning, you are no longer truly obese. That is, no matter how many pounds you are from your desired weight, if you have truly committed yourself to the bodily form you really want, your right brain and subconscious mind are now working toward that end. The physical manifestation is merely a matter of time.

RE-GROUPING

There is one final issue to discuss before I leave you to continue with your daily Reflective Relearning exercises and your resolve to obtain, maintain, and sustain your desired weight. I call it "getting your shift together," and it has to do with the attitudes and emotions of yourself and others as they affect your new determination to get and keep the bodily form you want.

Let's face it: None of us lives in a vacuum. In addition to all those old childhood tapes that tell us to "eat this and feel better" (Chapter 3) and those ever-present social tapes that confuse physical hunger with appetite and social expectations (Chapter 4), we must deal with the reactions of others — family, friends, and co-workers — to our increasingly trim bodies.

All of us must realize that our lives will alter, sometimes drastically, when we change our bodies. And some of us are surprised to find that, even though we have succeeded in reprogramming our thoughts and actions toward that final desired form, we didn't count on the possibility that our own personalities might change or that others might become threatened by us. When these new situations arise, we face the danger of returning to old, comfortable patterns of overeating. This is quite understandable: Who isn't at least a little afraid of navigating uncharted emotional waters and perhaps running aground in our relationships? Perhaps you would rather return to the safe port (as in "portly") of overeating?

Oh no you don't — you've come too far for that. Having gone through at least six weeks of Reflective Relearning, you are ready to venture into the open seas of your own and others' reactions to your changing body. Consider this chapter a navigational chart.

One of the best ways I've found to prepare people to "get their shift together" is to have them share with others their emotional experiences as they approach and maintain their desired weight. So in this chapter, I invite you to sit in on a typical group session as we discuss weight management. I'll play the role of leader, and you can be a new (silent) group member. The group, which is using a modified medical fasting program, is seated in a semicircle. Although you may not be following such a regime, you will hear the emotional challenges others face in changing their lifestyle adaptive patterns to reach a higher level of well-being. This should serve not only to make you aware that you are not alone, but also to provide strategies for dealing with your own experiences. So here goes.

Group Leader (Bobbe)   Good to see everyone here with smiling faces — you are smiling, aren't you? Right? Right! Okay, how is everyone doing? [Silence.] Please, not everyone at once. Yes, Ben?

Ben   Yeah, well, I'm not yet [he laughs] — how is it you put it? — "nonfood focused." Like, I thought about food all week this past week. I stayed on this diet — oops! I mean *program* — but I did miss eating. I'm not going to kid you about that one! [The group laughs.]

Bobbe I appreciate your honesty. Sure, you miss food. Remember, this is an artificial situation for you. This is a stopgap program to allow you to obtain your desired weight. It's a means to an end, not the end itself. Also, Ben, you've been on this program for only nine days, and your metabolism hasn't adjusted to the drastic change of taking in only 500 calories a day. Are you feeling okay physically?

Ben Yes, that part of me is okay. It's just that I can't seem to turn my head off. It wants to dwell on food like crazy.

Sue For me, the first two weeks were really hard, until my body adjusted to the idea of how it had to eat for a while. Honest, Ben, it gets better, and soon you'll learn to substitute other things for eating. Trust me, I never thought I'd say that! [The group laughs.] You can ask Bobbe here. I was a big complainer at first and thought I never would "get my shift together." I've been on the program for six months now — Reflective Relearning as well as the fast — and successfully gained my desired weight of 132 pounds. I've also been in this continuing support maintenance group for another four months. I may grow old here! Seriously, I know I need another few months to continue to learn my new lifestyle adaptive patterns.

Bobbe Thanks, Sue. I admire your willingness to be so candid. Can you put into words how you went about shifting your thinking patterns away from obsessive eating and toward other, more productive, thoughts? I think it would help Ben and the other new people who joined us tonight.

Sue Sure, if you don't mind my "soapbox speech." The truth is that when I first came here, less than a year ago, I had some pretty rotten habits. Like, I got up late, and dashed for work with a donut and coffee in the car. Then I smoked a cigarette and was ready to begin my day. Well, I've given up coffee and donuts for good, and Bobbe's on my tail now about my one last vice, smoking. I know, I know, I'm going to stop as soon as I convince myself I won't put on weight. And you know, I have no doubt that I will!

I guess the main turning point for me was to make myself stay in this group. Ask Bobbe. I copped out whenever I could. I realize now that I was afraid to look at myself objectively. I was embarrassed not only about my weight but also about my entire lifestyle. I finally committed to Bobbe to stick it out for one month. And here I am, still here nine months later — I could have had a baby by now! So for me, the commitment to look at myself was step number one.

Jack Yeah, me too. And step number two was to commit to making some major changes in my life. Both Sue and I decided in a group session about eight months ago to get up a half hour early and do some walking before we went to work. The group sure helped at the beginning. If I hadn't had to come here and report to Sue and the others how far I had walked each week, I know I'd have fallen off the wagon. But for me, getting moving was a major, even a giant, step.

Ben Do you still walk?

Jack Not only that, I do power-walking — you know, walking as fast as you can with your arms swinging hard. I don't want to jog, because I'm afraid it'll reinjure my old football knee. And I can tell you that not only do I feel good, I'm getting in shape so much faster than I ever thought possible, thanks to the group's support and their kicking me in the fanny every so often when I get discouraged.

Ben Well, I guess exercise probably is important, but I want to know how to get my mind off food. You guys are all way ahead of me. All I want to know is how to stop thinking about food all day long!

Sue Believe it or not, exercising will really help you take your mind off eating. After you walk for two or three miles doing the Reflective Relearning affirmations, you really aren't hungry afterward. I know — don't give me that look, Ben [she laughs]. I was ever so much more skeptical than you are. If only you could have known me before!

Karen She's right, Ben. All I can do is to tell you that the group works. Sue and a lot of us were pretty negative at the beginning and didn't really want to work for this weight stuff. I had the notion that I could just come here and "diet" like before and go about business as usual. But in this group, you don't. There's a lot of focus on moving, and on doing the Reflective Relearning time alone. You'll get to see a little bit about how it works tonight, when we do this technique in group at the end of the session. Sue and Jack and some of the oldtimers will tell you that if you think we were skeptical about exercising, you should have seen us when Bobbe started talking about doing Reflective Relearning during exercises. Talk about visions of wearing turbans and sitting on a hilltop in Tibet chanting weird mantras! But it's anything but that. Now we're all "hooked" on the Reflective Relearning method because it works.

Jack My wife had some concerns that doing Reflective Relearning might interfere with our religious beliefs, so I checked with our pastor, and he was one hundred percent in favor. In fact, he helped me learn to pray in such a way that I could use my Reflective Relearning time in combination with our way of praying. For me, it's been a lifesaver — and I mean that literally. I was killing myself with food, and my blood pressure was sky-high. Now it's back to normal, though I still have another twenty-three pounds to go till I reach my desired weight.

Bobbe Okay, I guess we're pretty much caught up on the nitty-gritty of what most of us want to share. Now I'd like to recap last week for those of us who weren't here. Would somebody like to volunteer?

Karen Well since I pretty well dominated the entire evening, I guess it's up to me to tell the new members what went on. I feel kinda strange, though, like I'm taking up even more time now.

Bobbe Feeling embarrassed?

Karen You got it. But one thing I've learned over the months of being here is that nobody is that unique, and we all have problems — 'scuse me, challenges — to meet in life. Bobbe's a great one for talking about upgrading problems to challenges. Problems have to be solved. Challenges need only be met.

Anyhow, last week I was sharing how my husband, Mike, is feeling threatened by my weight change. We've been married seventeen years, and I've never cheated on him, and he knows that in his heart. I weighed 186 when we were married, so I was no slim kid then. When I rocketed up to 256, I had to get the weight off, I was so miserable. And my last childbirth, five years ago, was the beginning of many physical complications for me. I hated myself and began to resent my family because they stayed skinny while I got fat. I took good care of Mike and the three kids and saw that they were fed right and the house was as perfect as I could keep it. That's a laugh! I was so careful that they ate well, yet I ate junk food myself. Typical, I guess, for an obsessive eater.

Well, Mike is feeling really threatened, like I'm about to have an affair or something. Now I weigh 142 and wear a size 12 — almost [she laughs] — and is he acting weird! Two weeks ago, when we went to bed, there was a candy bar (my favorite kind) under my pillow from Mike. He said he was giving me a reward for being so "noble." I was so miserable I burst into tears! He acted like he didn't know what was going on.

Bobbe Remember, Karen, he may not have consciously known what he was doing. Of course, he may have, but we must give him the benefit of the doubt.

Karen Yes, I know. But it's hard for me to believe he could be that dumb. I almost got hysterical that he could be so insensitive to my goal. Then I got mad. We've never had a fight like that before. I told him that if he didn't like the new me, he could just leave. He said it was fine with him. Anyhow, that's about where we ended group last week. Except that Bobbe stayed with me for a while alone and we talked about my feelings.

Bobbe Yes, and I feel that it's valuable for all of us to realize that some of us hit some very rough spots in the road when we change our bodies. Often, those around us become threatened or jealous.

Carolyn I have something along those lines to share, and maybe it could help with your situation, Karen. Mine may not be as serious as your problem (oops — challenge) with your husband, but it relates to how people around me reacted when I got to my desired weight.

I've been carpooling with the same four people for almost three years. We rotate times to drive and generally have a great time to and from work. Two of the group are men and two of us are women. We're all about the same age, give or take a few years. Anyhow, at the beginning of my fast, they were all supportive of my losing weight (pardon, *obtaining* my desired weight), although they were skeptical of the method I had chosen. My doctor had recommended it, and after investigating the alternatives, I agreed, so I didn't care what anyone said. Well, after a while, they all decided that I wouldn't die after all, and we settled back into our carpooling routine.

Anyhoo, we went to a play one Sunday afternoon, and the ones who were married brought their spouses, while one woman and I who were single went as a "couple." When one of the men's wives saw me, she was shocked at how "pretty" I was and made some crack about how she hoped I wasn't the last one her husband dropped off after work. I was crushed. She had always been so nice to me before. I felt that her joke wasn't ha-ha funny at all. I also realized that there was truth to it, because I saw Hal cringe. He just laughed, and I honestly felt that I would cry then and there. I knew she was jealous of me. I guess part of me might have felt flattered that she thought I was a threat to her marriage, but I don't work that way. She and Hal and I have been friends for three years, and I babysit for them — I even housesat for a month while they were out of the country. So I didn't know how to respond to her crack.

A little while later, it got even stickier. We stopped at a coffeehouse after the play and it was near dinnertime, so some of us decided to order dinner. I ordered a diet soda and had my packet of "stuff" to drink. She turned up her nose and said that it sure didn't smell good and that she didn't know how in the world I could do that to myself. I let it pass, but let me tell you, I was plenty angry and hurt and a lot of other feelings all rolled up into one little ball. Maybe Bobbe could help both Karen and me deal with these situations. What could we have said or done to feel better? I need to know ways of handling situations without my local anesthetic — food — to appease me. I swear to you, when I got home Sunday evening, for the first time since I've been on this program, I honestly wanted to eat.

Bobbe   Swallow your anger, maybe?

Carolyn   Probably.

Bobbe   Okay, let's see how we can "get our shift together" and handle these two situations. We'll discuss it and then do some role-playing. [The group moans.] Yes, it's embarrassing at first, but you must admit that when we do it, we all learn. [The group laughs.]
    It seems that both Mike and Hal's wife are feeling threatened. There's a fear element in operation here on both counts. What do these two people fear losing? Sure, they're afraid that their relationships with their "significant others" may change. Whenever any of us feel this, we get pretty touchy. We can all understand very well how Karen and Carolyn felt when these things happened to them.
    Now let's see if we can understand the other side of the coin. How do you suppose Hal's wife and Mike are feeling?

Jack   Probably afraid they'll lose a mate, or at least that their mate will be tempted, whereas before there was no threat, because fat people are considered fairly asexual — you know, kinda no gender. Suddenly your sex-stock goes way up when your body gets slender. So they're both probably not used to feeling this way toward these two formerly fat people.

Bobbe   Guess we'd better give you your honorary Ph.D. in psychology right now. That sounds pretty accurate to me. So let's see how we can help Karen and Carolyn respond to their situations.

Karen   Does this mean I have to role-play?

Bobbe   Yep, guess so. [They both laugh.]

Karen   I kinda thought that's what you had up your sleeve. Okay, let's go. Who do I play — me or Mike?

Bobbe   Why don't you play Mike and respond pretty much as you might expect him to respond, okay? I'll play your part and see if I can model some assertive behavior that will get your point across without injury to his high-level sensitivity. Remember, it has to be a win-win situation in order for it to work properly.

I'll start out by pretending to be you, Karen, and what I might say to Mike this evening is this: "Mike, I feel bad about our fight. I doubt that either of us meant what we said. How do you feel about it?"

Karen   I guess Mike would sulk first. He always does at first, then he settles down. So he would probably say something dumb, like, "Whatever you say — I don't know how I feel." See, that's why I get so mad at him. He cops out.

Bobbe   Don't let him cop out. Nicely nail him down with an answer something like this: "I can see you're still angry. Perhaps it's too soon to discuss it now. We can pick it up later, when you're more receptive to discussing it. I just wanted you to know that I feel bad about this and am open and willing to discussing what we can do to avoid another incident like that one. So let's try and talk about it later."

Karen   You mean, let him get off that easy? [The group laughs.]

Bobbe   For the time being. But you've made the initial step. Mike may be a slow starter and still need to brew some more before he commits to a response. Let's move it up a couple of days. If he hasn't brought it up then you can, by saying something to the effect that you really want to discuss the issue and come to some sort of resolution. Then you might just begin by stating how you felt that he was sabotaging your goal to be at your desired weight and that you really want him to know that you appreciate that he was attempting to reward you. Go further and explain that you truly are pleased that he thought about "rewarding" your nobility and that in the future you want him to reward you with nonfood items such as a flower on your pillow or a small gift.

Karen   I guess I should [she giggles] — I mean, I want — to give him the benefit of the doubt. I mean, if he really does want to reinforce and reward me for my "good behavior," I need to give him thanks for that.

Bobbe   That's right, and furthermore, you can retrain him on how to reward you nonnutritionally by making a straightforward statement about how you want to be rewarded. Remember, Mike can't read your mind any more than you can read his. It's your job to tell him assertively what you want and how you want to be rewarded.

Karen   This is true. I know it, but when I feel that he deliberately tempted me with candy to get me fat again, I get so empty inside that I really feel I could die.

Bobbe   Yes, your *feelings* are the key point here. I want to get into how you can understand these feelings. He needs to know that he may have a hidden agenda here to sabotage your goal. He might not be conscious of what he's doing. First, I want to point out your use of the words "get so empty inside."

Karen   What?

Bobbe   You said that you get so EMPTY inside.

Karen   I did? [The group members nod their heads and laugh.] No kidding? I didn't even hear that. Boy, what a tale that tells, huh?

Bobbe   The Freudians would say that was a "Freudian slip." And these slips are oftentimes right on in reference to our true feelings. Karen, could it be that subconsciously, whenever you feel rejected, you translate it into "feeling empty"?

Karen　I guess the proof of the pudding [here she laughs and the group joins her at the usage of food as a metaphor for her feelings] — What can I tell you? There it is. Not only do I use words like "feeling empty," I use "pudding" as an example! [Karen and the group laugh heartily.]

Bobbe　How true of many of us, Karen. You're in good company here! How many of us have delegated our feelings to mistranslations of food thoughts?

Ben　As you were talking, Karen, I realized that all this week I was feeling deprived and that the words running through my head were literally that I had an empty, lonely feeling, as though I had just lost a good friend. I know that sounds really crazy, but it's the way it seemed to me.

Bobbe　Not crazy at all, Ben. Many of us befriend food as a source of comfort when we feel "empty" or alone or deprived. So when this "reward" is withheld, there's a sense of grief. There's a real sense of loss.

Ben　You don't know how good it is to have someone understand these feelings! I mean, the average guy off the street would send for the wagon and the men in white coats if I let these feelings out. It's worth a lot to me to have people like you guys here tell me that I'm not some kind of nut.

Sue　Ben, I, too, have had to realize that I had to go through a real grieving period when I wouldn't let myself binge in the evenings like I used to. I've even sat in the kitchen and cried because I wanted to eat — at least a part of me still wants to eat — and I know I will *not* succumb to this. I've kept my forty-seven pounds off for five weeks now. I know that isn't long for most people, but for me it's a world record.

Bobbe really helped me understand that any feeling of loss results in a grieving period. I used to think "grief" was when your best friend died — you know, really heavy-duty stuff. Now I see that there is a series of "minigriefs" in my life, and in the lives of others as well. I allow these feelings to come to me, and I no longer make myself "wrong" for genuine feelings. If I really, truly miss eating my half gallon of double-chocolate-chip ice cream, then there's a sense of loss. My intellectual side won't permit me to indulge in this process any longer, but the good ol' emotional side still remembers how good it felt. Good, that is, for the first few minutes after I ate the ice cream. Now I tell myself to stop and remember the afterthoughts — the recriminations, the self-hating. Do I really choose this for myself? Do I really need to suffer? No, no, NO!

Bobbe Thanks, Sue. I want to underline the use of the word "choose." We talked at length a few days ago about the importance of learning to choose and choose again. We have the right to make new choices as we go along and to do this in a manner that is supportive of our greater good. Just because we've made choices in the past that were nonsupportive doesn't mean we're chained to these choices. In the past, Sue, you chose to eat ice cream when you felt "empty" of love and acceptance. Today you choose other things. Will you tell us what you choose now?

Sue Sure. I learned through the group here that it's okay to feel the loss of my food-friend. I meant what I said about sitting in the kitchen and crying. I still do, once in a while. Thank goodness it gets easier. I occasionally sit there crying and being on the "pity pot" for as long as it takes for me to sense the loss. The important thing to remember is that after I go through this crying or bereavement, then I ask myself, "Do you *choose* to eat ice cream? If you really consciously choose to eat it, then go ahead." For me, this is the key point. Then I make a *conscious choice*. It's what Bobbe refers to as "delayed gratification." My long-term goal of being a size 10 is more important to me than eating ice cream because my boyfriend didn't call as he promised.

Bobbe Excellent point, Sue. Your eating ice cream really didn't punish your boyfriend. It ended up punishing you.

Sue You got that one right! I can remember eating ice cream out of the carton over the kitchen sink — anyone here relate? [The entire group chuckles and nods in agreement.] I can vividly recall thinking, "I'll show you" as I ate. Talk about dumb!

Bobbe Seems dumb now, but at the time you were doing it, you were attempting to soothe your feelings of rejection. Remember, for many of us, being fat is faulty problem solving. You attempted to meet the challenge of feeling rejected by filling the "empty" sensation with food, which also served to "show him."

Sue It's true that Steve is the first one who complained when I put on weight. His comments about my being "broad in the beam" weren't exactly subtle. So I guess my eating was in punishment of him. [She begins to laugh.] As a matter of fact, I remember telling myself that because he didn't see me tonight, when he does see me, he'll see more of me than he ever dreamed possible. He'll see lots and lots of me! [The group laughs.]

Bobbe Great. It's important for all of us to keep our sense of humor. And it's supportive to know that everyone in this group laughs *with* the person sharing and not *at* him. We've all been in the same boat at some time in our lives.

   The important thing to remember is that even though some of our bingeing seemed bizarre and nonsensical at the time we did it, in reality the behavior was an attempt to solve a problem. That's what we must realize. Now we're free to make new choices about meeting the challenges of life.

   Sue, we got sidetracked. How do you now meet these challenges in nonnutritional ways?

Sue Oh yeah. I got so carried away by telling about how I showed Steve my rebellious side that I forgot. Well, I let myself grieve and cry and be on the pity pot until, frankly, I get tired of it all. Then I ask myself if I really want the food. If I make a conscious choice to eat it, then I do. If not, I choose to do something good for my body. Lately, I've been rewarding myself by doing some yoga postures and then doing my nails or working on my knitting. I'm making Steve a ski scarf — I may hang him with it if he doesn't call me! [Everyone laughs.] Seriously, though, I do tell him now to can the cracks about my being "broad in the beam." I told him a few days ago that I would no longer tolerate his verbal abuse. He said I was making a mountain out of a molehill. I said maybe I was, but it was important to me that he stop. He just mumbled something and ignored it. But so far he hasn't made passing potshots at me about my weight since then.

Bobbe   Sure feels good to say how we really feel rather than "swallow our anger," doesn't it? [The group members nod.]

Jack   I would like to emphasize something to the new people, especially Ben, since he has expressed concern about being "food focused." As I mentioned earlier, I'm really excited about my change in attitude after beginning my power-walking. In the beginning, I told myself that I would do it, but I doubted that my attitude toward food would change. I sorta did what Bobbe calls "faking it till you make it" — head trips, I admit, but for me it worked. After about two weeks of power-walking every day, I noticed that I felt much better psychologically. My attitude toward food *did* change. It seemed that my dwelling on what to eat next diminished. I know that some of the literature says that regular exercise releases some hormones in the body — endorphins — which help the person have a sense of well-being.
 Believe me, I had to literally force myself to get up one hour early and walk in the dark and the cold. I wanted to cop out, but my pact with the group kept me going. Besides, I didn't want to look foolish in front of the group and have some "girl" show me up, as chauvinistic as that sounds. So this incentive was enough to keep me going until my subconscious mind gradually took over the idea of power-walking, and it became a habit. A pleasant habit, I might add. So, all I want to say is, keep a positive outlook and learn to "fake it till you make it," because you *will* make it.

Bobbe   Thank you, Jack. We all remember being the new kid in the group, and anything we can do to inspire the rest of the group is very helpful. Your point about "faking it till you make it" is valid. You see, we've discussed the workings of the conscious and subconscious minds enough to know that the affirmations we make during our daily Reflective Relearning exercises are eventually assigned to the automatic, subconscious mind. We find ourselves thinking, "Of course I'll go for my walk — what else?" It becomes a natural part of our daily routine, like brushing our teeth and making the bed.

Now, since our time is almost up for tonight, I would like everyone to get comfortable, and I'll lower the lights and we'll do our Reflective Relearning affirmations. Remember, these are best repeated to yourself on your daily walks, swims, or while doing yoga or any other form of activity your choose for yourself.

[The group leader now leads the group in a Reflective Relearning exercise and assists them in their affirmation:

"I WILL ALLOW MYSELF TO OBTAIN, MAINTAIN, AND SUSTAIN MY DESIRED WEIGHT OF _____ POUNDS BY _____ ."]

FULFILLED, NOT FILLED FULL: RITA

I want to leave you with a case history to finally illustrate how we can deal with the tumultuous emotions that may accompany a weight change. Let's see how one formerly fat person has dealt with her emotions in new ways, which in turn helps her to keep her weight at her desired level. She is Rita, a schoolteacher who lives alone. She has taught in the same school for fourteen years, and she loves her job. She is truly dedicated to giving each child in her fifth-grade class individual attention and the love he or she is entitled to receive.

Rita began getting fat when she was a freshman in college. She found herself dating less and less and eating more and more. This didn't really bother her, however, since she was totally dedicated to her studies. After graduation, she landed the job she still holds. Subsequently, she went back to school and received her master's degree in education, and she is currently going to night school for her doctorate in elementary education.

Rita has dated very little during her fourteen years of teaching school and honestly says that it didn't bother her much — until recently, when she learned that she was developing diabetes and her physician convinced her that she had to drop some weight. She went on a modified medical fast at her doctor's suggestion. At this point, she weighed 306 pounds, the most she had ever weighed.

As she made rapid progress toward obtaining her desired weight, her personality began to change, and she believed that it was changing for the worse. She reported feeling irritated with her peers and even with the children at times. She felt herself wanting to "tell people off." It was in a support group that Rita began to experience feelings of deep anger at the people with whom she worked, especially the school principal. These feelings confused her, and she finally made some appointments with me to clarify what was happening. As her anger began to surface, she became increasingly anxious and started sleeping poorly. She had been extremely faithful to her fasting program during the six weeks she had been on it. She had eaten nothing but the assigned food supplement and had lost about thirty-five pounds. She reported that those with whom she worked, including her male principal, were very complimentary and supportive of her program. Why, then, was she so angry? Sometimes on her way home from work, she would become full of rage and then burst into tears and feel quite shaky and faint. Her physician ruled out any physical complications from her modified medical fast, so she decided to enter into psychotherapy.

After only two sessions, Rita began to understand what was happening to her. Like all of us, Rita had trouble seeing what was obvious to others: She was releasing the anger that she had held inside for fourteen years. All those years, "good ol' Rita" could be counted on to volunteer for extra playground duty, to bake birthday cakes for everyone on the staff, and to take on the "challenging" children without complaint. Now she was beginning to see more clearly that she had been "swallowing her anger" and paying a high price in order to be considered a "nice girl." She also saw that although she hadn't been obese as a child, she had

had the same feelings of needing to win favor from parents and other authority figures. She had been the one in the family who was most congenial.

Now, as she began to inch her way toward her goal weight, Rita began to feel differently about being taken advantage of. During one session, I asked her to close her eyes and rest for a moment, and then, with eyes still closed, to speak the names of the people with whom she was angry. She began speaking softly, but within five minutes she was shouting. She was shocked and embarrassed (and afraid the therapists in the next room would hear her). I asked Rita to go home and find a way to get in touch with her anger *safely,* and to do some physical activity, such as walking, to release these old emotions. Emotions and feelings are always buried alive, never dead, and we often think that these old feelings are gone, only to find one day that they have resurfaced.

When Rita came back the next week, she reported that when she had arrived home from work the day following her last session, she had felt the tears about to flow. She went out to her backyard and happened to pick up an orange that had fallen from her tree. She glanced up and saw the aluminum shed she used for storage, and the next thing she knew, she was throwing oranges like crazy! Each orange was another peer. She laughed when she told me that she had the most dented-up shed in her neighborhood.

With only a few more private sessions and continued group sessions, Rita learned to release her anger at these people and to focus on where the real anger was. She learned quickly to understand her anger and realized that she did not have to act with hostility. She was, naturally, angry at herself for having given so much and received so little, and she gradually learned to understand why and to forgive herself and others with whom she worked. She learned that her congenial behavior was a coping skill that she had used to make her feel that she was a part of the staff, even though she was the only really obese person there. As her self-esteem began to rise with her movement toward her desired weight, she began to experience her anger and thus began to release it.

Like Rita, we need to experience our emotions — and the

emotions of others — before we can begin to deal with them in ways that do not threaten our well-being or our goals. When correctly understood, these emotions can lead to growth. Rita's anger really got her attention and forced her to look at her behavior over the past fourteen years. She soon got the message and accepted her anger as the learning experience it was. She no longer felt the need to throw oranges, and she also saw her personality changing dramatically.

One day, Rita even attended a Board of Education meeting, which she admitted she would not have done a few weeks before, and complained about an issue that had been bothering her for eight years. She started saying "no" more often and allowed others to bake the birthday cakes. She even reported that the staff had given her a giant birthday "cake" of her own — a pyramid of diet colas with a big bow on top, plus a large card of congratulations.

When Rita hears messages playing in her head to eat, she says "cancel" out loud now. She walks three miles every day after work and feels wonderful. As she walks, she repeats to herself her Reflective Relearning affirmations about her weight. She also practices role-playing in her car on the way to work. It is still difficult for her to say no, particularly to her principal, but as she role-plays various situations, it becomes easier for her to talk with him and assert herself. She plays both parts, anticipating what he might ask of her. In general, she feels much better about herself and her life and even admits that she does want to date when her weight is where she wants it to be. Her group is encouraging her to begin to attend singles events. So far, she has gone to only one, but even though she danced just one dance, she came home delighted with herself.

Rita also says "next time" to herself when she makes a mistake or gives in to unreal demands. She realizes that in the past she felt so insecure that she would do anything to gain favor. Now she realizes that as she changes her behavior and the old tapes in her head, she will still fall back into old patterns from time to time. She accepts this, and when she "slips," she says to herself, "Next time, I'll . . . ". What's more, her diabetic condition is much improved, and her blood pressure is normal for the first time in many years.

When asked how she knows that she'll keep the weight off, Rita replies, "I walk three miles every day now, and as of next month, that goes up to four miles and finally to five miles when I get to 200 pounds. Then I'll start exercise classes — very moderate, but a start. At 150 pounds, I'll start my full exercise program, coupled with my power-walking. I can truthfully say that I will never be fat again, and I can also swear to you that I will do my Reflective Relearning every day of my life for at least ten minutes a day."

Rita says that this is the first time in her life that she has known for sure that she will not regain her weight. She has some practical tools to help her when she is tempted to overeat — tools that include building a better plan when she's "blown it" ("Next time, I'll . . . "), getting on a regular exercise program, and correcting herself when she hears her subconscious mind telling her that she's hungry. When this happens, she says aloud, "Rita, what do you *really* want?" She gets her answer, and she acts on it.

Rita is a wonderful example for all of us. She has learned to take care of her needs by fulfilling them directly rather than filling herself full. She has learned to replace the old food = comfort images of her right brain with new ones equating comfortable emotions with nonfood rewards. And she has used her left brain to *consciously* become aware of her urges and control them.

Thank you, Rita, and all of you who have allowed me to share your stories in this book, for setting an example for the millions who share your challenge. Through your success, we know that there are others like us who have faced and met the weight challenge.

And to you, my readers, a last word: Remember that no "diet book" can ever replace your own determination and your right to make choices. Through these choices, you *can* achieve everything you want — not only in your weight, but in all areas of life!

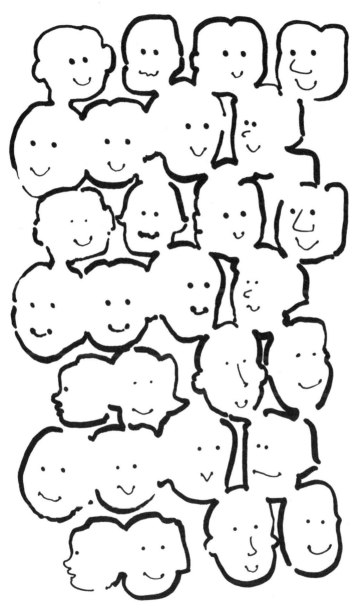

Through these choices you can achieve everything you want —
not only in your weight but in *all* areas of life.

Appendix I

Our Two Brains:
History and Suggested Reading

As I pointed out in Chapter One, the evidence that each of us has two brains in one has been around for a long time. In 1836, Marc Dax, a country doctor, reported what seemed to be a significant relationship between brain-damaged patients suffering speech loss and the side of the brain on which the damage appeared — the left. Now, the idea that specific areas of the brain are associated with specific functions (sight, smell, moving the left pinkie, and so on) was not new; in fact, the notion that speech resided in the frontal lobes of the brain had gained some acceptance among scientists. What was new was the idea that the brain's two halves, right and left, controlled separate functions.

Dax's radical suggestion was ignored. He died in 1837, and his observations received little attention until the early 1860s, when the French surgeon Paul Broca again noticed the association between speech loss and left-hemisphere brain damage. Broca also noticed that left-brain-damaged patients were often paralyzed on one side of their bodies — the right, or the side opposite to the damaged hemisphere. Indeed, it is a well-known fact today that the two halves of the brain control movements and sensations on the opposite sides of the body. Stroke patients make this graphically evident: Those with damaged left brains suffer speech loss and paralysis on the right side; those with damaged right brains suffer no loss of speech but may show other deficiencies (difficulty finding their way around the hospital, for example), as well as the predictable paralysis on the left side.

By the end of the nineteenth century, scientists had begun to accept the notion of a "leading" or "dominant" side of the brain — which, for the vast majority of right-handers and at least half of all left-handers, proves to be the left hemisphere. It is interesting that the discovery that verbal functions are seated in the left brain led to terms such as "leading hemisphere" and "cerebral dominance." These terms assume the superiority of that part of the brain which controls the understanding and production of language. This is not suprising. Our verbal, logical abilities are so important to socialized human existence that we would have a hard time surviving without them.

Nevertheless, the special functions that seem to be the domain of the "minor" (usually right) side of the brain also began to emerge. Indeed, the originator of the "leading hemisphere" idea, the British neurologist John Hughlings Jackson, noted in 1868 that "if . . . it should be proven by wider experience that the faculty of expression [speech or verbal ability] resides in one hemisphere, there is no absurdity in raising the question as to whether perception — its corresponding opposite — may be seated in the other." Jackson was suggesting that *both* sides of the brain — the right as well as the left — have their special functions, both of which are essential to full human existence.

In 1935, T. Weisenberg and K.E. McBride performed extensive tests on more than two hundred patients. These tests revealed, predictably, that the seat of verbal ability lies in the left hemisphere of the brain. They also found, however, that right-brain-damaged patients were significantly less able to perform tasks that called on nonverbal abilities — the ability to assemble puzzles or complete missing parts of patterns or figures, for example — which required an understanding of spatial relationships.

In the early 1940s, William Van Wagenen, a New York neurosurgeon, performed the first split-brain operations on humans in order to relieve epileptic seizures. Van Wagenen undertook this as a last-resort surgery in response to evidence that cutting the *corpus callosum* (the major band of nerve fiber connecting the two halves of the brain) could alleviate epileptic seizures. Although the operations did not produce the hoped-for results, they did open the way for others to investigate the functions of the corpus callosum — and hence the two cerebral hemispheres.

In the 1950s, Ronald Myers and Roger Sperry discovered that severing the corpus callosum of a cat caused visual information available to one side of the cat's brain to be unavailable to the other side. Subsequent tests of such animals revealed further differences, adding to our current understanding of the subtle, complex, yet distinct, abilities possessed by the two hemispheres. The real breakthrough in understanding the dual functioning of the brain came in the 1960s, when Sperry and his students Michael Gazzaniga and Jerre Levy began their historic split-brain experiments. In these experiments, the researchers were able to test separately the thinking abilities of two surgically separated halves of the human brain. They found that each half has its own separate train of conscious thoughts and its own memories. Even more important, they found that the two sides of the brain think in fundamentally different ways: While the left brain tends to think in words, the right brain thinks directly in sensory images.

Currently, scientists believe that each hemisphere contributes certain specialized functions to overall human behavior. The most obvious and clear-cut differences concern verbal (or language) abilities. In the vast majority of people, the ability to produce and understand speech depends heavily on the left side of the brain. The right side seems to excel in spatial abilities: The recognition of spatial relationships that allows us to put on our clothes, move from room to room, recognize faces — in short, the ability to respond to, form, and store pictorial images that mean something to us.

There are other dramatic differences between our two brains. The right brain seems to control a good portion of our musical abilities: Left-brain-damaged patients, while often unable to speak, can sing familiar songs; their right-brain-damaged counterparts can speak but are unable to sing. Right-brain-damaged patients can recognize people's faces (even though they may not be able to say "Hi, Joe!"); left-brain-damaged patients have difficulty doing so, unless they learn "cues" (such as the presence of a moustache) to help them differentiate one person from another. When an image of a spoon was flashed to the visual space perceived by the right brain, a person could identify the object as a spoon only by picking up an actual spoon with her left hand (remember, the right brain can recognize spatially related contours and also controls motor activity of the left side). When asked to say what she saw,

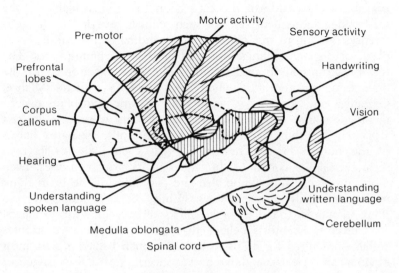

Lateral view of the brain showing some major structures and functions.

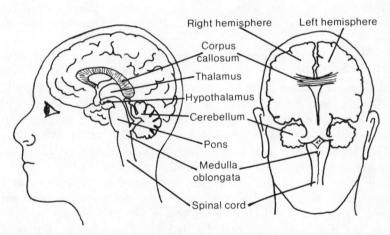

The entire nervous system is essentially bisymmetric. The central nervous system does not physically separate until the thalamus.

however, she protested that she saw nothing, or only a flash of light, since her left brain (where the word-symbol "spoon" is stored) was deprived of the visual information.

One of the most intriguing differences in right- and left-brain abilities has to do with emotions. Patients who have sustained damage to the right hemisphere are often unable to interpret or respond to the "body language" of others, as expressed in a raised eyebrow, an angry tone of voice, an open-armed welcome. Moreover, these patients have difficulty expressing emotion; they seem to have lost touch with their feelings.

There are various schools of thought concerning to what, exactly, we can attribute these differences in the functions of our two brains. Recent investigation suggests that hemispheric specialization is not an all-or-none proposition. Unless damage to one side of the brain is dramatic and pervasive, the other side can, in time, compensate for the lost abilities; that is, each hemisphere seems capable of handling many different kinds of tasks. Often, however, the two sides of the brain seem to differ in both their approach and their efficiency. It's not enough to say, for example, that the right brain is the "music maker," because many of the more analytical functions connected with composing and performing music seem to be associated with the left brain.

There are, however, certain characteristics that align themselves with one or the other hemisphere. These characteristics have been summarized by Sally P. Springer and Georg Deutsch in their excellent book, *Left Brain, Right Brain*, and are reproduced here.

Left Hemisphere	*Right Hemisphere*

PROCESSES*

Verbal	Nonverbal, visuo-spatial
Sequential, temporal, digital	Simultaneous, spatial, analogic
Logical, analytic	Gestalt, synthetic
Rational	Intuitive
Western thought	Eastern thought

Left Hemisphere	*Right Hemisphere*

DICHOTOMIES

Intellect	Intuition
Convergent	Divergent
Intellectual	Sensuous
Deductive	Imaginative
Rational	Metaphoric
Vertical	Horizontal
Discrete	Continuous
Abstract	Concrete
Realistic	Impulsive
Directed	Free
Differential	Existential
Sequential	Multiple
Historical	Timeless
Analytic	Holistic
Explicit	Tacit
Objective	Subjective
Successive	Simultaneous

SOURCE: Sally P. Springer and Georg Deutsch, *Left Brain, Right Brain* (New York: W.H. Freeman and Company, ©1981), pp. 185–186. Reprinted with permission.

---

* Springer and Deutsch note that these processes are ordered, from top to bottom, according to the extent of empirical evidence available for each pair. Hence, the verbal/nonverbal dichotomy is substantiated by the most empirical evidence; the Western/Eastern dichotomy is most speculative.

BIBLIOGRAPHY & SUGGESTED READING

For those who want to read more about right-brain functioning and research, a list of resources is given below in alphabetical order by author. Several papers listed are quite technical and specialized, so the books that I consider especially interesting and readable are marked with a large asterisk to make them easier to find.

Akelaitis, A. J., W. Risteen, R. Herren, and W. Van Wagenen. "Studies on the Corpus Callosum: III. A Contribution to the Study of Dyspraxia in Epileptics Following Parial and Complete Section of the Corpus Callosum." *Archives Neurological Psychiatry* 47 (1942), pp. 971–1008.

* Arguelles, Jose, and Mariam Arguelles. *Mandala*. Boulder, CO: Shambhala, 1972.

Bakan, Paul. "Hypnotizability, Laterality of Eye-Movements and Functional Brain Asymmetry." *Perceptual and Motor Skills* 28 (1969), pp. 927–932.

Bakan, Paul. "The Right Brain Is the Dreamer." *Psychology Today* (November 1976), pp. 66–68.

Bell, E., and L.M. Karnosh. "Cerebral Hemispherectomy: Report of a Case Ten Years After Operation." *Journal of Neurosurgery* 6 (1949), pp. 285–293.

* Blakeslee, Thomas R. *The Right Brain*. Garden City, NY: Doubleday, 1980.

Bogen, Joseph E. "The Other Side of the Brain: I. Dysgraphia and Dyscopia Following Cerebral Commissurotomy." *Bulletin of the Los Angeles Neurological Societies* 34 (1969), pp. 73–105.

Bogen, Joseph E. "The Other Side of the Brain: II. An Appositional Mind." *Bulletin of the Los Angeles Neurological Societies* 34 (1969), pp. 135–162.

Bogen, Joseph E., and Glenda M. Bogen. "The Other Side of the Brain: III. The Corpus Callosum and Creativity." *Bulletin of the Los Angeles Neurological Societies* 34 (1969), pp. 191–217.

Bogen, Joseph E., R. DeZure, W. D. Tenhouten, and J. F. Marsh. "The Other Side of the Brain: IV. The A/P Ratio." *Bulletin of the Los Angeles Neurological Societies* 37 (1972), pp. 49–61.

Bogen, Joseph E., and Michael S. Gazzaniga. "Cerebral Commissurotomy in Man: Minor Hemisphere Dominance for Certain Visuospatial Functions." *Journal of Neurosurgery* (1965), pp. 394–399.

Bogen, Joseph E., and P. S. Vogel. "Cerebral Commissurotomy in Man." *Bulletin of the Los Angeles Neurological Societies* 29 (1962), pp. 169–172.

* Bry, Adelaide, with Marjorie Bair. *Directing the Movies of Your Mind.* New York: Harper & Row, 1978.

Caramazza, A., J. Gordon, E. Zurif, and D. DeLuca. "Right-Hemispheric Damage and Verbal Problem-solving Behavior." *Brain and Language* 3 (1976), pp. 41–46.

Dacey, Rob. "Inside the Brain: The Last Great Frontier." *Saturday Review* (August 9, 1975), p. 13.

Deglin, Vadim. "Split Brain." *The UNESCO Courier* (January 1976), pp. 5–32.

Deikman, Arthur J. "Biomedical Consciousness." *Archives General Psychiatry* 25 (1971), pp. 481–489.

Dimond, S., and J. G. Beaumont. "Experimental Studies of Hemisphere Function in the Human Brain." In S. Dimond and J. G. Beaumont (eds.), *Hemisphere Function in the Human Brain.* New York: John Wiley, 1974.

Dimond, S., L. Farrington, and P. Johnson. "Differing Emotional Response from Right and Left Hemispheres." *Nature* 261 (1976), pp. 690–692.

Doyle, Stuart. "Evolution and Lateralization of the Brain: Concluding Remarks." *Annals of the New York Academy of Science* 299 (1977), pp. 477–499.

* Edwards, Betty. *Drawing on the Right Side of the Brain.* Los Angeles: J. P. Tarcher, 1979.

* Ferguson, Marilyn. *The Brain Revolution.* New York: Bantam, 1975.

Franco, Laura. "Hemispheric Interaction in the Processing of Concurrent Tasks in Commissurotomy Subjects." *Neuropsychologia* 15 (1977), pp. 707–710.

Franco, Laura, and Roger W. Sperry. "Hemisphere Lateralization for Cognitive Processing of Geometry." *Neuropsychologia* 15 (1977), pp. 15, 107–114.

Galin, David. "Implication for Psychiatry of Left and Right Cerebral Specialization." *Archives General Psychiatry* 31 (October 1974), pp. 572–583.

Garrett, Susan V. "Putting Our Whole Brain to Use: A Fresh Look at the Creative Process." *Journal of Creative Behavior* 10 (1976), pp. 239–249.

* Gawain, Shakti. *Creative Visualization.* Mill Valley, CA: Whatever Publishing, 1978.

Gazzaniga, Michael S. "The Split Brain in Man." *Brain and Consciousness* (August 1967), pp. 118–123.

* Gazzaniga, Michael S. *The Bisected Brain.* New York: Appleton-Century-Crofts, 1970.

Gazzaniga, Michael S. "One Brain — Two Minds?" *American Scientist* (May/June 1972), pp. 311–317.

Gazzaniga, Michael S. "Review of the Split Brain." *Journal of Neurology* 209 (1975), pp. 75–79.

Geschwind, Norman. "Specialization of the Human Brain." *Scientific American* 241 (September 1979), pp. 180–199.

Goldstein, Marvin N., Robert J. Joynt, and Ronald B. Hartley. "The Long-term Effects of Callosal Sectioning." *Archives of Neurology* 32 (1975), pp. 52–53.

* Hampden-Turner, Charles. *Maps of the Mind.* New York: Macmillan, 1981.

Hardyck, C. "Individual Differences in Hemispheric Functioning." In H. Whitaker and Whitaker (eds.), *Studies in Neurolinguistics* (Vol. 3). New York: Academic Press, 1977.

Hoppe, Klaus D. "Split Brain — Psychoanalytic Findings and Hypotheses." *Journal of the American Academy of Psychoanalysis* 6, No. 2 (1978), pp. 193–213.

* Jaynes, Julian. *The Origin of Consciousness in the Breakdown of the Bicameral Mind.* Boston: Houghton Mifflin, 1976.

Kimura, D. "Left-Right Differences in the Perception of Melodies." *Quarterly Journal of Experimental Psychology* 16 (1964), pp. 355–358.

Krashen, Stephen D. "The Major Hemisphere." *UCLA Educator* 17 (Spring 1975), p. 17.

Krashen, Stephen D. "Cerebral Asymmetry." In H. Whitaker and Whitaker (eds.), *Studies in Neurolinguistics* (Vol. 2). New York: Academic Press, 1977.

Ledoux, Joseph E., Gail L. Raisse, Sally P. Springer, Donald H. Wilson, and Michael S. Gazzaniga. "Cognition and Commissurotomy." *Brain* 100 (1977), pp. 87–104.

Lee, P., R. Ornstein, D. Galin, A. Deikman, and C. Tart. *Symposium on Consciousness.* New York: Viking, 1976.

Levy, Jerre. "Cerebral Asymmetries as Manifested in Split-Brain Man." In M. Kinsbourne and A. Smith (eds.), *Hemispheric Disconnection and Cerebral Function.* Springfield, IL: Charles C. Thomas, 1974.

Levy, Jerre. "Psychobiological Implications of Bilateral Asymmetry." In S. Dimond and J. G. Beaumont (eds.), *Hemisphere Function in the Human Brain.* New York: John Wiley, 1974.

Levy, Jerre, Robert D. Nebes, and Roger W. Sperry. "Expressive Language in the Surgically Separated Minor Hemisphere." *Cortex* 7 (1971), pp. 49–58.

Ornstein, Robert E. "The Split and Whole Brain." *Human Nature* 1 (May 1978), pp. 76–83.

Penfield, W., and R. Lamar. *Speech and Brain Mechanisms.* Princeton, NJ: Princeton University Press, 1959.

Pribram, Karl H. "Hemispheric Specialization: Evolution or Revolution?" *Annals of the New York Academy of Science* 299 (1977), pp. 18–21.

Restak, Richard M. "The Brain." *The Wilson Quarterly* (Summer 1982), pp. 89–113.

Sage, Wayne. "The Split Brain Lab." *Human Behavior* (June 1976), pp. 25–28.

Samples, Robert E. "Are You Teaching Only One Side of the Brain?" *Learning* (February 1975), pp. 25–28.

* Samuels, Mike, and Nancy Samuels. *Seeing with the Mind's Eye: The History, Techniques and Uses of Visualization.* New York: Random House, 1975.

Schwartz, G. E., R. J. Davidson, and F. Maer. "Right Hemisphere Lateralization for Emotion in the Human Brain: Interactions with Cognition." *Science* 190 (1975), pp. 286–288.

Selnes, Ola Arvid. "The Corpus Callosum: Some Anatomical and Functional Considerations with Special Reference to Language." *Brain and Language* 1 (1974), pp. 111–140.

Sperry, Roger W. "The Great Cerebral Commissure." *Scientific American* (January 1964), pp. 42–52.

Sperry, Roger W. "Brain Bisection and Mechanisms of Consciousness." In John C. Eccles (ed.), *Brain and Consciousness Experience.* New York: Springer-Verlag, 1966.

Sperry, Roger W. "Split-Brain Approach to Learning Problems." In G. C. Quarton, T. Melnechuk, and F. C. Schmitt (eds.), *The Neurosciences: A Study Program.* New York: Rockefeller University Press, 1967.

Sperry, Roger W. "Hemisphere Deconnection and Unity in Conscious Awareness." *American Psychologist* 23 (1968), pp. 723–733.

Sperry, Roger W. "Left Brain, Right Brain." *Saturday Review* (August 9, 1975), pp. 30–33.

Sperry, Roger W. "Some Effects of Disconnecting the Cerebral Hemispheres." Nobel Prize Lecture, December 8, 1981.

Sperry, Roger W., E. Zaidel, and D. Zaidel. "Self-Recognition and Social Awareness in the Disconnected Minor Hemisphere." *Neuropsychologia* 17, pp. 153–166.

* Springer, Sally P., and Georg Deutsch. *Left Brain, Right Brain.* San Francisco: W.H. Freeman and Company, 1981.

Tucker, D. M. "Lateral Brain Function, Emotion, and Conceptualization." *Psychological Bulletin* 89 (1981), pp. 19–46.

Zaidel, Dahlia, and Roger W. Sperry. "Memory Impairment After Commissurotomy in Man." *Brain* 97 (1974), pp. 263–272.

Zaidel, Dahlia, and Roger W. Sperry. "Some Long-term Motor Effects of Cerebral Commissurotomy in Man." *Neuropsychologia* 15 (1977), pp. 193–204.

Zaidel, E., D. W. Zaidel, and R. W. Sperry. "Left and Right Intelligence: Case Studies of Raven's Progressive Matrices Following Brain Bisection and Hemidecortication." 1981.

* Zdenek, Marilee. *The Right-Brain Experience.* New York: McGraw-Hill, 1983.

Appendix II

Nutrition Basics: Starting A New Eating Program

This is not a book about nutrition or dieting, as I have stated again and again. The focus of this book is on how to eat — in fact, how to *think*, through Reflective Relearning, about eating — in order to get and keep your desired weight. No amount of information on nutrition, and certainly no diet, will work for us until we change our attitudes toward food, and come to believe that we can and will get the bodily form we want. That is what Reflective Relearning is all about.

Yet, as you engage in the Reflective Relearning process and begin to obtain, maintain, and sustain your desired weight, you will find that your eating patterns are changing, too. At that time, you may wish to investigate (or reacquaint yourself with) some of the basics of nutrition so that you can plan a sensible, safe, and satisfying new program for getting the nutrients your body needs.

This appendix is *not* a diet. It simply offers some guidelines for developing a healthy eating program, lists some basic nutritional facts, and refers you to several books on nutrition.

WHAT TO EAT? FINDING A NEW APPROACH

Before selecting a new eating program, the first thing you must do is consult your physician. He or she is aware of your medical history and any conditions that may limit or modify the foods you consume. In consultation, the two of you can develop a nutritional plan that will suit your individual needs.

After discussing your weight goal with your physician, you

may also wish to consult a nutritionist — one who is licensed to do nutritional counseling. Ask your doctor to refer you to one. There are also a number of reputable organizations devoted to sensible, safe weight reduction, including Weight Watchers, TOPS, Overeaters Anonymous, and Diet Center. These and similar organizations, upon your doctor's approval, can be good sources of healthy eating programs. Many also offer regular meetings, which provide invaluable moral support and social contact.

The Basic Nutrients: Where To Find Them

The following is a list of the nutrients essential to the healthy functioning of the human body, and the foods that provide them:

Protein: Meat, fish, poultry, eggs, milk, cheese, legumes, nuts (and nut butters), wheat germ, brewer's yeast.

Unsaturated Fats: Vegetable and most nut oils, salad dressings, mayonnaise, nuts and nut butters, margarine.

Complex Carbohydrates: Flours, grains, fruits, vegetables.

Calcium: Milk and milk products, dark green leafy vegetables, canned sardines and salmon, almonds, sesame seeds, soybeans and soy products, oats, egg yolks.

Iron: Lean and glandular meats, chicken (dark meat), shellfish, legumes, dried fruits (especially raisins, prunes, and apricots), egg yolks, whole grain products.

Sodium: Prepared (canned or frozen) foods, salt-water fish, pickles, milk, cheese, eggs, baking soda and powder, fresh vegetables (especially carrots, beets, spinach, and celery).

Potassium: Bananas, oranges, avocados, vegetables (especially potatoes, winter squash, tomatoes, and leafy greens).

Magnesium: Bananas, whole grain products, legumes, milk, dark green leafy vegetables, nuts.

Phosphorus: Whole grain products, bran, cheese and milk, legumes, eggs, meats, peanuts and peanut butter.

Iodine: Iodized and sea salt, kelp and other seaweed, saltwater seafoods.

Zinc: Beef, eggs, liver, herring, oysters, brown rice, oatmeal, sunflower seeds, kelp and other seaweed, carrots, peas.

Vitamin A: Deep-yellow and orange fruits and vegetables (especially carrots, sweet potatoes, apricots, winter squash, pumpkin, and cantaloupe), yellow corn and cornmeal, whole milk, cream, butter, whole milk cheeses, liver, dark green leafy vegetables (such as broccoli, escarole, spinach), and tomatoes.

Thiamine: Pork, heart, kidneys, liver, legumes, whole grain products, wheat germ, brewer's yeast, peanuts and peanut butter.

Riboflavin: Meats (especially liver, kidneys, and heart), milk, cheese, dark green leafy vegetables, brewer's yeast, whole grain products.

Niacin: Lean meat (especially liver, poultry and fish), legumes, whole grain products, wheat germ, brewer's yeast, nuts.

Vitamin B-6:   Chicken, fish and shellfish, meats, egg yolks, legumes, whole grain products, dark green leafy vegetables, potatoes, bananas, prunes and raisins, brewer's yeast, nuts.

Folacin: Liver, dark green vegetables, legumes, nuts.

Pantothenic Acid: Organ meats, eggs, bran, peanuts, oats, whole wheat and wheat germ, pork, beef.

Vitamin B-12: Meats (especially glandular meats), milk and cheese, fish, eggs (especially egg yolks), wheat germ, brewer's yeast, kelp and other seaweed.

Vitamin C: Fruits Fruits (especially citrus, cantaloupe, and strawberries), vegetables (green and red peppers, tomatoes, potatoes cooked in skins, raw cabbage, brussels sprouts, and broccoli).

Vitamin D: Fortified milk, egg yolks, fish-liver oils (and sunshine, too).

Vitamin E: Vegetable oils, wheat germ, whole grain products, peanuts, dark green leafy vegetables.

These facts should serve your figure well. Once you have "digested" this information, you can begin to build a wise nutritional program. The specific *types* and *proportions* of foods to eat in order to stay healthy while you approach your desired weight are, I repeat, matters for you and your physician to decide.

RATING THE DIETS

Then there are the diets, which I have deliberately avoided discussing in the main text of this book — except to say that even the most sensible of them will not work unless and until you are committed to obtaining, maintaining, and sustaining a healthy, desirable bodily form.

But let's face it: None of us (especially those of us who are substantially overweight) can avoid hearing about the many diets out there. They are hyped in newspapers, on television, and in book ads. And there are some diets that meet good nutritional standards and may be right for you — but *only* with the approval of your physician and *only* after you have committed yourself to obtaining, maintaining, and sustaining your desired weight.

Never plunge "mouth long" into that latest diet bestseller or summer slimdown program without first consulting your doctor and then totally committing yourself to a long-term process. If you are quick to grasp at the illusion that there are only "ten days to a new you," you are letting yourself in for intense disappointment at best (probably accompanied by more self-destructive bingeing); at worst, you could be playing havoc with your health.

Let's assume, then, that you are planning that all-important discussion with your physician about your desire to obtain and maintain a lower weight. I can recommend three publications on diets and dieting to start you off: The United States Senate's *Dietary Goals for the United States* (1977), Iva Bennett and Martha Simon's *The Prudent Diet* (1973), and Theodore Berland's *Rating the Diets* (1983). *Dietary Goals* can be obtained through U.S. Government Printing Office bookstores, which exist in most major cities in the United States. (You can also write directly to the Washington, D.C., office: North Capitol and H Streets NW; WDC 20401). Both *Dietary Goals* and *The Prudent Diet* are based on the best medical and nutritional findings, and list protein, carbohydrates, and some fats as essential nutrients (warning, however, that excessive *saturated* fats endanger the heart and blood vessels).

In *Rating the Diets*, Theodore Berland rates more than one hundred diets according to a star system. Four stars indicate the "best" diets: those providing adequate protein, no more than 30% of their calories in fats (predominantly unsaturated fats), and a prominent portion of carbohydrates, with very little sugar. A three-star rating indicates a somewhat deficient diet: one that may omit a particular food group and emphasize another, or one that may not properly balance proteins, fats, and carbohydrates, for example. A two-star rating identifies the high-protein diets and warns that extraordinarily high intake of protein may also result in high intake of cholesterol, which can pose a threat to people with kidney or heart trouble. A one-star rating indicates a "fad diet:" one that may have a few saving graces, but, although not dangerous, is basically foolish. The no-star diets are unrealistic and downright dangerous to your health.

I recommend all three of these publications to those of you considering embarking on any of the myriad diets now available.

Rating the Diets will help you, along with your physician, to choose an appropriate nutritional plan for you.

A SELECTED BIBLIOGRAPHY

Aside from the publications listed above, there are numerous books and articles on nutrition, fitness, and weight management. I have selected a few to list here, some designed for general readers and some for those who "get into" the subject enough to desire more extensive information.

Abraham, Sidney. "Weight by Height and Age for Adults 18–74 Years, United States, 1971-74." In U.S. Department of Health, Education and Welfare, *Vital and Health Statistics: Series 11, Data from the National Health Survey*, no. 208 (DHEW Publication no. PHS 79-1656). Washington, D.C.: U.S. Government Printing Office, 1979.

Andersen, Marianne S. "The Treatment of Obesity by Hypnotherapy." *Dissertation Abstracts International* 41, 8 (1981). (Order #8100631)

Bailey, Covert. *Fit or Fat?* Boston: Houghton Mifflin, 1977.

Bennett, Iva, and Martha Simon. *The Prudent Diet.* New York: David White, 1973.

Bennett, William, and Joe Gurin. *The Dieter's Dilemma.* New York: Basic Books, 1982.

Berland, Theodore. *The Fitness Fact Book.* New York: Almanac, 1980.

Berland, Theodore. *Rating the Diets.* Skokie, IL: Consumer Guide Publications International Ltd., 1983.

Briggs, George M., and Doris H. Calloway. *Nutrition and Physical Fitness.* Philadelphia: W. B. Saunders, 1979.

Bruch, Hilde. *Eating Disorders.* New York: Basic Books, 1973.

Bruno, Frank J. *Think Yourself Thin.* Los Angeles: Nash, 1972.

Chaney, Margaret S., Margaret L. Ross, and Julia C. Witshci. *Nutrition.* Boston: Houghton Mifflin, 1979.

Christians, George F. *The Compulsive Overeater.* New York: Doubleday, 1978.

Dawber, Thomas Royle. *The Framingham Study: The Epidemiology of Atherosclerotic Disease.* Cambridge, MA: Harvard University Press, 1980.

Deri, Susan. "A Problem in Obesity." In Arthur Burton and Robert Harris (eds.), *Clinical Studies of Personality.* New York: Harper & Brothers, 1955.

Deutsch, Ronald M. *Realities of Nutrition.* Palo Alto, CA: Bull, 1976.

Duffy, William. *Sugar Blues.* New York: Warner Books, 1976.

Dusky, Lorraine, and J. J. Leedy. *How to Eat Like a Thin Person.* New York: Simon & Schuster, 1982.

Edelstein, Barbara. *The Woman Doctor's Diet for Women.* Englewood Cliffs, NJ: Prentice-Hall, 1977.

Edwards, Sandra. *Too Much is Not Enough.* New York: McGraw-Hill, 1981.

Fleck, Henrietta. *Introduction to Nutrition.* New York: Macmillan, 1976.

Goldstein, Yonkel. "The Effect of Demonstrating to a Subject that She is in a Hypnotic Trance as a Variable in Hypnotic Interventions with Obese Women." *International Journal of Clinical and Experimental Hypnosis* 24, 1, pp. 15–23.

Goodhart, Robert S., and Maurice E. Shils. *Modern Nutrition in Health and Disease*. Philadelphia: Lea & Febiger, 1973.

Guthrie, Helen A. *Introductory Nutrition*. St. Louis: Mosby, 1979.

Hamilton, Eva May, and Eleanor Whitney. *Nutrition Concepts and Controversies*. St. Paul, MN: West Publishing Company, 1979.

Hoffman, Lieselotte. *The Great American Nutrition Hassle*. Palo Alto, CA: Mayfield, 1978.

Howe, Phyllis S. *Basic Nutrition in Health and Disease*. Philadelphia: W. B. Saunders, 1971.

Jacobson, Michael F. *Eater's Digest: The Consumer's Factbook of Food Additives*. New York: Doubleday, 1976.

Jolliffe, Norman. "The Prudent Man's Diet." *House Beautiful* (January 1961).

Katch, Frank I., and William D. McArdle. *Nutrition, Weight Control, and Exercise*. Boston: Houghton Mifflin, 1977.

Klingman, Mildred. *The Secret Lives of Fat People*. Boston: Houghton Mifflin, 1981.

Labruza, Theodore P. *Food for Your Well-Being*. St. Paul, MN: West Publishing Company, 1977.

Labruza, Theodore P. *The Nutrition Crisis: A Reader*. St. Paul, MN: West Publishing Company, 1975.

Labruza, Theodore P., and A. Elizabeth Sloan. *Contemporary Nutrition Controversies*. St. Paul, MN: West Publishing Company, 1979.

Lappe, Frances Moore. *Diet for a Small Planet* (revised ed.). New York: Ballantine, 1982.

Leisy, James. *Calories In, Calories Out*. Battleboro, VT: Stephen Greene Press, 1981.

LeShan, Eda. *Winning the Losing Battle*. New York: Crowell, 1979.

Lindner, Peter G. "Overeaters Anonymous: Report on a Self-Help Group." *Obesity/Bariatric Medicine* 3 (1974), pp. 134–137.

Lindner, Peter G., and George L. Blackburn. "Multidisciplinary Approach to Obesity Utilizing Fasting Modified by Protein-Sparing Therapy." *Obesity/Bariatric Medicine* 5 (1976), pp. 198–216.

Livingston, Carole. *I'll Never Be Fat Again!* Secaucus, NJ: Lyle Stuart, 1980.

Mayer, Jean. *Overweight — Causes, Cost, and Control*. Englewood Cliffs, NJ: Prentice-Hall, 1968.

Mayo Clinic Diet Manual. Philadelphia: W. B. Saunders, 1971.

Millman, Marcia. *Such a Pretty Face: Being Fat in America*. New York: Norton, 1980.

Mitchell, Helen S., Henderika J. Rynbergen, Linnea Anderson, and Marjorie V. Dibble. *Nutrition in Health and Disease*. Philadelphia: J. B. Lippincott, 1976.

Morehouse, L.E., and A. T. Miller, Jr. *Physiology of Exercise*. St. Louis: Mosby, 1967.

Mott, Thurman, Jr., and Joan Roberts. "Obesity and Hypnosis: A Review of the Literature." *American Journal of Clinical Hypnosis* 22 (July 1979), pp. 3–7.

"New Weight Standards for Men and Women." *Statistical Bulletin of the Metropolitan Life Insurance Company* 40 (November/December 1959), pp. 1–4.

Orbach, Susie. *Fat is a Feminist Issue.* New York: Paddington Press, 1978.

Osman, Jack D. *Thin from Within.* New York: Hart, 1976.

Overeaters Anonymous. *Compulsive Overeating and the OA Recovery Program.* Torrance, CA: Overeaters Anonymous.

Physical Fitness Calculator. Washington, D.C.: U. S. Government Printing Office, 1975.

Pike, Ruth L., and Myrtle L. Brown. *Nutrition: An Integrated Approach.* New York: John Wiley, 1975.

Prince, Francine. *Diet for Life.* New York: Bantam Books, 1982.

Pritikin, Nathan. *The Pritikin Permanent Weight-Loss Manual.* New York: Grossett & Dunlap, 1981.

Pritikin, Nathan, and Patrick M. McGrady, Jr. *The Pritikin Program for Diet and Exercise.* New York: Grossett & Dunlap, 1979.

"The Prudent Diet: Vintage 1973." *Medical World News* 10 (August 1973), pp. 34–44.

Rechtshaffen, Joseph S., and Robert Carola. *Dr. Rechtshaffen's Diet for Lifetime Weight Control and Better Health.* New York: Random House, 1980.

Rubin, Theodore Isaac. *Forever Thin.* New York: Bernard Geis, 1970.

Smith, Nathan J. *Food for Sport.* Palo Alto, CA: Bull, 1976.

Smith, R. Philip. *The La Costa Diet and Exercise Book.* New York: Grossett & Dunlap, 1977.

Solomon, Neil, and Evalee Harrison. *Doctor Solomon's Proven Master Plan for Total Body Fitness and Maintenance.* New York: G. P. Putnam's Sons, 1976.

Stanton, H.E. "Weight Loss Through Hypnosis." *American Journal of Clinical Hypnosis* 18 (October 1975), pp. 94–97.

Stanton, H. E. "Fee-Paying and Weight Loss: Evidence for an Interesting Interaction." *American Journal of Clinical Hypnosis* 19 (July 1976), pp. 47–49.

Stare, Frederick J. "Nutritional Facts and Fictions as They Relate to Health and Disease." American Society of Bariatric Physicians. Annual Obesity and Related Conditions Symposium, Las Vegas, Nevada, October 29, 1982.

Stare, Frederick J., and Margaret McWilliams. *Living Nutrition.* New York: John Wiley, 1977.

Stuart, Richard B. *Act Thin, Stay Thin.* New York: Norton, 1978.

Stuart, Richard B., and Christine Mitchell. "Self-Help Groups in the Control of Body Weight." In Albert J. Stunkard (ed.), *Obesity.* Philadelphia: W. B. Saunders, 1980.

Stuelke, Richard G. *Thin for Life.* New York: Baronet, 1977.

Stunkard, Albert J. "The Success of TOPS, a Self-Help Group." *Postgraduate Medicine* (May 1972), pp. 143–147.

Stunkard, Albert J. *The Pain of Obesity.* Palo Alto, CA: Bull, 1976.

Stunkard, Albert J. *I Almost Feel Thin!* Palo Alto, CA: Bull, 1977.

Stunkard, Albert J., Harold Levine, and Sonija Fox. "Study of a Patient Self-Help Group for Obesity." Presented at the 122nd annual meeting of the American Psychiatric Association, Miami, Florida, May 1969.

Ulene, Art. *Feeling Fine.* Los Angeles: J. P. Tarcher, 1977.

U.S. Department of Agriculture/Health and Human Services. *Nutrition and Your Health: Dietary Guidelines for Americans.* Washington, D.C.: U.S. Government Printing Office, 1980.

U.S. Senate Select Committee on Nutrition and Human Needs. *Dietary Goals for the United States.* Washington, D.C.: U.S. Government Printing Office, 1977.

Whitney, Eleanor, and May Hamilton. *Understanding Nutrition.* St. Paul, MN: West Publishing Company, 1977.

Williams, Sue Rodwell. *Nutrition and Diet Therapy.* St. Louis: Mosby, 1977.

Willis, Judith. "About Body Wraps, Pills and Other Magic Wands for Losing Weight." *FDA Consumer* 16 (November 982), pp. 18–20.

Young, Charlotte. "Planning the Low-Calorie Diet." *American Journal of Clinical Nutrition* 8 (December 1960), p. 898.

Index

Use This Handy Order Form for *SPECIAL DISCOUNT*
on Hunter House **Family & Health Books**

CHARTING YOUR WAY THRU' PMS by Virginia M. Fontana et. al.
A woman's health book and planning guide. Charting your menstrual symptoms is the *only* reliable way to diagnose PMS, and this book helps you do it.
Soft Cover   64 pages   Illustrated $2.95

DRINKING PROBLEMS = FAMILY PROBLEMS by Marie-Louise Meyer, R.N.
The problem drinker affects all those around him. This book discusses the choices that must be made, the changes to carry through to regain control of your life.
Hard Cover   256 pages $12.95

EXCLUSIVELY FEMALE: A Nutrition Guide for Better Menstrual Health by Linda Ojeda, Ph.D. Nutrition and diet can help relieve the symptoms of premenstrual syndrome and other causes of menstrual discomfort. Includes a nutrient guide for adult women.
Soft Cover   160 pages $5.95

GETTING HIGH IN NATURAL WAYS An Infobook for Young People of All Ages by Nancy Levinson and Joanne Rocklin, Ph.D. Being high is a natural state — *and we don't need drugs to get there.* A vitally important book for our times.
Soft Cover   112 pages $6.95

HELPING YOUR CHILD SUCCEED AFTER DIVORCE by Florence Bienenfeld, Ph.D.
A guide for divorcing parents who want — and need — to make this time as safe as possible for their children. Filled with practical strategies for resolving conflicts.
Soft Cover   224 pages   Illustrated $9.95

MENOPAUSE WITHOUT MEDICINE by Linda Ojeda, Ph.D.
Preparing for a healthy menopause can never begin too early. Ojeda's natural approach focuses on nutrition, physical conditioning, beauty care, and psychological health.
Hard Cover   320 pages   Illustrated $17.95

NOT ANOTHER DIET BOOK: A Right-Brain Program for Successful Weight Management by Bobbe Sommer, Ph.D. Right brain techniques to gain control of your weight, self-image, *and* your life. Includes a six-week program to obtain and maintain the desired weight.
Hard Cover   256 pages $15.95   32 illustrations

NUTRITION AND YOUR BODY by Benjamin Colimore, Ph.D., and Sarah Colimore.
Comprehensive and easily read scientific information on how nutrients work in the body and why we need them; with practical advice, recipes, meal planners, and tips that make the difference.
Soft Cover   260 pages $9.95

ONCE A MONTH: The Original Premenstrual Syndrome Handbook by Katharina Dalton, M.D. The first book — and still the best — to explain clearly the symptoms, effects and complete treatment of Premenstrual Syndrome. By the acknowledged pioneer in the field.
Soft Cover   256 pages   3rd Edition $8.45

PMS: PREMENSTRUAL SYNDROME A Book for Teenage Women, Their Friends and Families by Gilda Berger. The first need is proper information, and this book will help young women through their encounters with PMS.
Soft Cover   96 pages $6.95

RAISING EACH OTHER: A Book for Parents and Teens by Jeanne Brondino and the Parent/Teen Book Group. Honest talk from both generations about freedom, privacy, trust, responsibility, drugs, drinking, sex, other vital issues.
Soft Cover   128 pages $7.95

Prices Subject to Change Without Notice
See Over for Ordering and Discounts

Add postage and handling at $1.50 for one book and $0.50 for every additional book. Please allow 6 to 8 weeks for delivery.

PLEASE PRINT:

Name _____

Street/Number _____

City/State _____ Zip _____

PLEASE SEND ME:

CHARTING YOUR WAY . . . . _____ @ $ 2.95 _____

          Pack of 10 . . . . _____ @ $25.00 _____

DRINKING PROBLEMS = FAMILY PROBLEMS . . . . . _____ @ $12.95 _____

EXCLUSIVELY FEMALE . . . . _____ @ $ 5.95 _____

HELPING YOUR CHILD SUCCEED . . . . _____ @ $ 9.95 _____

GETTING HIGH IN NATURAL WAYS . . . . _____ @ $ 6.95 _____

MENOPAUSE WITHOUT MEDICINE . . . . _____ @ $17.95 _____

NOT ANOTHER DIET BOOK . . . . _____ @ $15.95 _____

NUTRITION AND YOUR BODY . . . . _____ @ $9.95 _____

ONCE A MONTH . . . . _____ @ $ 8.45 _____

PMS INFOBOOK . . . . _____ @ $ 6.95 _____

RAISING EACH OTHER . . . . _____ @ $ 7.95 _____

                                                TOTAL $_____

          DISCOUNT AT _____ %   **LESS $(_____)**

          TOTAL COST OF BOOKS $_____

          California Residents add 6% Sales Tax $_____

          Shipping & Handling $_____

          TOTAL AMOUNT ENCLOSED $_____

     ☐ **Money Orders**   ☐ **Check**

     ☐ **Check here to receive our catalog of books**

Please complete and mail to:
HUNTER HOUSE INC., PUBLISHERS
PO Box 847, Claremont, CA 91711, USA

If you don't use this offer — give it to a friend!

DR. BOBBE SOMMER
Helps you take control of your weight, your self-image, and your life:

NOT ANOTHER DIET BOOK A Right-Brain Program for Successful Weight Management
Additional copies of this book are available direct from the publisher. Use the handy order form.   *Soft Cover   240 pages $8.45*

NOT ANOTHER DIET PLAN
Formerly titled, "Leaving Your Fat Behind." A set of four cassettes that take you step by step through Dr. Sommer's techniques of Reflective Relearning to reprogram attitudes about food, about eating — and about yourself!   *Four Audio Cassettes $49.95*

GETTING YOUR SHIFT TOGETHER
"We do not WORK on transforming our lives, we merely follow the necessary steps to become receptive and the transformations follow." This four-cassette program contains the "mechanics" of how to allow transformations to come into your life.   *Four Audio Cassettes $49.95*